Hold Your Prem

a workbook on skin-to-skin contact
for parents of premature babies

This book is dedicated to our children, Rebecka, Simon and
Emma, who give us our greatest joy! My husband and I
have both had wonderful parents who gave us love, fun and
a secure base of trust to build our lives. We have tried to do
the same for our children.

Dear Sylvia!
This works.

NILS

5/7/10   UCSF $15

First Published in South Africa 2010
by
New Voices Publishing
Cape Town, South Africa
www.newvoices.co.za

First Edition February 2010 in paperback

ISBN - 978-1-920411-15-2

DISCLAIMER.

Mother-infant skin-to-skin contact is a safe place for caring for newborn and premature babies - but should only be practiced safely, and under the supervision and responsibility of health professionals. Authors accept no liability for any adverse events. The information and advice expressed in this book are believed to be accurate, and based on the best evidence available. This book is NOT a substitute for current care in any way; premature newborns should be cared for by health professionals practicing evidence based medicine.

The publisher is not responsible for errors or omissions.

Hold Your Prem

a workbook on skin-to-skin contact
for parents of premature babies

by Jill Bergman, BA HDE

with
Dr Nils Bergman, MB ChB, DCH, MPH, MD

CONTENTS

HOW TO USE THIS BOOK

This is a <u>practical workbook</u>

It has been written to help Mums and Dads in the scary situation of expecting or having a premature baby (or just "prem").

It gives <u>key information</u> needed to understand the prem and the NICU (the Neonatal Intensive Care Unit).

It describes <u>practical steps</u> and tasks that help parents be central in the team that is helping their prem.

This book is a tool to encourage and empower parents.

To Mum and Dad:

This book is organised into chapters for you to look up easily. Though they have an order, you can read them in any order you like.

If your prem is already born, then the <u>most</u> important information you will find quickly and easily on **BLUE PAGES**. These are "front page summaries" of what you want to know, and you can start by reading only these.

You will then know where to look for more details, in the pages that follow.

Read the other sections as you need them.

If you are likely to have a premature baby, try to read this book before your baby is born. Getting the first hours of life right will help you and your prem.

This is a workbook, so you will see spaces where you can write things down. For example, your own prem's details, treatment, and some of your own reactions. There are suggestions of things to do or observe. You will find this helpful in this difficult time. I encourage you specially to work through the chapter on "Emotions". Seeing these things written down will help you face them. This is important for you to be able to better help your prem, and cope better for yourself!

Some information may seem new or surprising to you. Your NICU staff might also be surprised by what is here! However, every statement has firm scientific evidence behind it. A number inside brackets in the text, e.g. (2), refers to the "Fine Print Page" at the end of each chapter. This has comments by Dr Nils Bergman, and the scientific references. The fine print page is for you if you want more detail, but it is also addressed to your doctor or nurse who can look up the evidence for what is being said.

I welcome your feedback and suggestions to make this book more helpful.

Jill Bergman

jill@kangaroomothercare.com

(February 2010)

INTRODUCTION

Many parents come to me after a talk on prematurity and say

"If only I'd known...I would have done things differently."

Any mother or father who has sat watching their little prem in an incubator struggling to breathe knows that feeling of utter helplessness and despair, and the agony of leaving their tiny baby so alone in hospital. But there is an alternative! It is "skin-to-skin contact".

HOLD YOUR PREM

This short book is for you parents who find yourselves in the scary, confusing situation of having a premature baby. Some babies may go to the Neonatal Intensive Care Unit (NICU) if they are sick or need special care. All of the information given is valid for these babies and their parents too.

There are thousands of parenting books in the bookstores. There is as much advice out there as there are women and grannies in the world! But almost all of the advice given is from the parents' perspective! Yes, parents like to have their sleep and their "well-behaved baby" and will buy the books that promise them what they want. Unfortunately, this is very often not what the baby needs and wants.

This is a baby-centred book, based on the baby's basic biological needs, both physical and emotional. In particular, it speaks for the premature newborn, who cannot speak for herself.

This is a workbook and has been written to help you to help your baby. It gives simple information and practical things that you can do to be central in the team that is helping your premature baby.

There are so many different terms: premature infant, baby, preemie, prem, etc; I will use the simplest, prem. I will also write as if the baby is a girl, as there are many cultures that do not value girls as highly as boys. Every baby is a gift!

Some information may seem new or surprising to you, but every statement has firm scientific evidence behind it. A number inside brackets in the text, e.g. (2) refers to the "Fine Print Page" with comments and references at the end of each chapter. The fine print page is for you if you want more detail, but it is addressed to your doctor or nurse who can look up the evidence for what is being said.

There are some strong statements in this book. It is not my intention to offend, but to challenge parents and staff members to consider the recent research showing what is best for the baby. All the evidence proves that the mother of the newborn is vitally important for her child's optimal development.

I also do not mean to make you as parents feel guilty if you were not allowed to give the best care to your baby. I want you to have the evidence you need to empower you, and the tools to do all that you can to make up for your baby's rough start. No-one else and no artificial incubator can provide anything like Mum's best care. The prem's own mother's milk provides food specific to the baby's needs. No artificial milk formula can ever come close!

Personal testimony of a mother at International KMC Workshop

"The instinct of a mother to hold and care for her baby is primordial and primitive and an overwhelmingly powerful feeling."

Jane Davis, Bogota, Dec 1998

It is natural to want to be with your baby.

It is right.

You, Mum, must trust your instinct of love and nurture.

The bond between the newborn child and mother is vital and forms the basis for all relationships later. Why has this changed so much lately? What will the impact of this be on the present and future generations?

> **Humans are mammals. This means that they breastfeed their infants with their own milk.**

The fierceness with which she protects her young is the measure of how good an animal mother is. It is her natural maternal instinct and it is needed for the survival of her baby.

It will be your natural instinct to protect your baby too. But often in our technological age you as parents may feel paralysed and disempowered by the sight of all the machinery in a NICU. You may feel worry, fear, confusion and uncertainty. You may feel very vulnerable at this stage as you want the best for your baby and you may think that an incubator is what your baby needs. The machines may be needed but you are needed even more!

As a new parent of a prem, you need to know that you are not alone, that there are many other new parents who are feeling the same worry and trauma as you are (about one in 8 babies in the world is born prematurely). Each mother and father will have different feelings, each hospital and clinic situation will be different; each premature baby will have her own unique complications of being born too early.

The technology that we have in the modern world is amazing and wonderful, and your baby should have access to all the technology that she needs to survive. The younger she is, perhaps the more machinery is needed. But we also need to understand what modern neuroscience is proving time and again; what the prem baby needs most can best be provided by the mother.

This is written for all parents of all prems, whether in a high-tech NICU or places with less resources, because the babies' basic biological needs are the same. In places that do not have access to first world technology, giving skin-to-skin contact alone may save the baby's life (1). In a NICU where people have access to incubators and all of the machines needed, knowing this information will help them to give all of the technological support needed, but in the right place: on the mother's chest.

Interestingly many cases are recorded of very small babies who were not expected to survive who were put on their mothers' chest. These babies started to dramatically improve and even grew faster than the incubator babies! This convinced hospitals to do skin-to-skin contact. Susan Ludington-Hoe starts her book with one such example (2).

Parents may say that in their hospital doing skin-to-skin contact at birth is not possible, and that the doctors and nurses insist on "stabilising" the baby first. Firstly, there is no technical definition for what a "stable" baby is. Secondly, there is solid scientific evidence that shows that a baby becomes more stable more quickly on her mothers chest (3). You may need to challenge the systems and ask for your baby to get all the technical support she needs while she is on your chest.

<u>**Never separate mother and baby.**</u>
This is the key to the best development for the premature baby.
The science behind this shows that:
1.   **the mother provides all the sensory stimulation needed for the brain of the baby to grow;**
2.   **skin-to-skin contact is the best way to provide this ideal care.**
Technology should be added; it is not a substitute for the mother.

This book will help you understand the technology your baby needs and give you practical ways to help your prem's development so that later problems are reduced as far as possible.

If you are likely to have a premature baby, try to read this before your baby is born to get those first hours right. This will make things easier for you and your baby. If your baby is already in a NICU, you may not have much time; read the first page of each chapter. Read the other sections as you need them.

It is my hope and prayer that this information will lessen the stress of having a premature baby and that it will help you and your prem to cope better.

THE FIRST FEW HOURS

▶ Skin-to-skin contact should start at birth, or as soon after that as possible.

▶ This is for all babies, and even more so for prems.

▶ This helps them stabilise their heart, breathing and temperature best.

Mum, ask for your naked baby to be put on your naked chest straight after delivery in the labour ward (4).

She can be dried off and both of you can be covered together. All the tests and assessments can be done while she is on your chest.

She should stay with you like that for at least the first hour; she should not be taken away or bathed during that time. It is very likely that your baby will smell and make her own way to your nipple and try to latch on (5). Encourage her. Your baby should not be suctioned at this time as it will disturb her suckling reflex (6).

As your baby is born, she needs you, her mother.

You provide the sensations which make your baby feel safe; this in turn makes her stable.

The brain of the baby is developing from very early in pregnancy. During the last third of the pregnancy, the brain development is huge. This usually happens inside the mother, and this is what the baby expects biologically. If your baby is born premature, this brain development will be occurring in the NICU which is NOT ideal, and we need to minimize the shock for her.

Skin-to-skin contact provides the biologically expected stimulation to wire the brain in the best way possible. The skin-to-skin contact between mum and baby is the way that the mother's 'autonomic nervous system' (ANS) tells the baby's ANS how to regulate.

The brain is stimulated by sensations. Sensations from the mother are good and reassuring. They make the brain develop. As time passes, new sensations stimulate new parts of the brain to connect. This brain-wiring depends on mother's presence. I shall explain this in detail in a later chapter.

AT BIRTH YOUR BABY NEEDS and expects to

1. feel your skin against hers, keeping her warm and you holding her tight;

2. smell you (that is her first sense to develop);

3. hear your voice and heartbeat (she's heard them for months – both will soothe her);

4. see you! (she knows what a face is and looks for you);

5. taste your breast and later your milk.

SENSATIONS THAT WIRE THE BRAIN

SEES Mum's eyes · Ear HEARS Mum's voice · SMELLS Mum's milk · MOVES with Mum · TASTES Mum's milk · Back FEELS Mum's arm holding · Hand TOUCH Mum's skin · Skin-to-skin CONTACT · WARMED on Mum's front

The technology that separates a mum and her prem deprives the baby's brain of her basic needs.

An "incubator" is what is used to hatch chickens! The American name "Isolette" shows that the baby is isolated from her mum and dad. This is not a good thing – she needs you, her parents.

Skin–to–skin contact with your baby

0–90 minutes after birth	is critical for her best brain development, physically and mentally.
0–6 hours after birth	will help her cardio-respiratory (heart and breathing) systems to stabilize, physically.
6–24 hours after birth	helps the baby to get into a stable feeding pattern and sleep cycling.
12 hours to 8 weeks after birth	is essential for attachment and bonding.

If you are reading this and your baby is already a few days old, you do not need to feel guilty; start skin-to-skin contact straight away to help you and your little one to bond closely and to help breastfeeding. She needs you to hold her close for weeks for her brain to grow properly. If you can only start this late, just continue longer!

As your baby is born

Your baby has been born too early and she is called a premature baby (prem). She has had a rough start; her brain is not fully developed, her lungs may not be ready for breathing air, her sight and hearing are extra sensitive, and her skin is extra fragile.

As you look at her you may think that she is far too tiny and delicate to touch, and you may worry whether she will survive. She may need machines to help her breathing, tubes in her nose or mouth for feeding, and heel pricks for blood tests. Nothing "nice" has happened to your baby. The doctors and nurses will do all they can to help her fight for her life, but you need to know that she needs you, her mum and dad more than anything else in the world.

You may wish that it was different, but I want to encourage you by showing that there is so much that you can do in these first hours and days of her life that may even mean life or death for her. Most of all, it is the long-term quality of life which is at stake. Helping her to be close to you will give her good physical and mental health now and

for her whole life.

Your baby has been safe inside you for months, held close, warm and safe, hearing your heart beat and your voice. Your body has given her everything that she needs. Now that she is out in the big wide world too early, your job is to carry on giving her everything that she needs. Yes, you still can! She may need machines, but here are some practical things that you can do.

Practical:

It is very important to know that your tiny baby is YOUR tiny baby and she needs you. She longs to be held in skin-to-skin contact (SSC), on your chest. This is her safe place. Ask the nurses to dry her gently and put her naked on your naked chest as she is born, and to cover both of you with a soft cloth and a blanket.

Your chest is the best place for your baby to adjust to life.

On your chest: **your baby will stay warmer and calmer,**
cry less, and
have better blood sugars

compared to being swaddled or put in a crib or an incubator (4).

Premature babies cannot control their own body temperature and they lose heat very quickly. Do not let her be taken and washed as this will make her temperature swing badly. The nurses and doctors can do all their tests while she is safely and peacefully on your chest. Your hands are there to help hold her still.

Separation from you will cause your baby stress; gently and firmly insist that she stays with you.

Ask that she is left on your chest for the first hour at least. Hold her as much as you can, for as long as you can. When she cries, the stress hormones in her body make her heart beat faster which sends more blood around the body. This uses up energy, and she needs all the energy she has to grow. If a tiny prem is stressed then her heart rate and blood pressure increases, this may cause the tiny blood vessels in the brain to burst (a brain bleed). Keep her calm in skin-to-skin contact to avoid this.

If your baby is extremely small, she may need CPAP, (continuous positive airways pressure) which is a way of providing extra pressure to each breath. If she is not managing on CPAP, she may need surfactant, or ventilation, and then the doctor may need to separate her from you. Your baby may also have medical conditions that require management that is not practical to do on your chest. When there are such good reasons for separating you and your baby, then you should agree, but you have the right to a proper explanation! You can then start working on a plan to get together again as soon as possible.

You may feel overwhelmed – that's OK. It is a whole new role being a mother and it is a huge shock that your baby has been born early.

Skin-to-skin Contact (SSC), cuddling and bonding help you and your baby to relate to each other better. Snuggling at birth gives you and your baby the best start for breast-feeding, and helps longer-term breast feeding. These first few hours are important for "Self-Attachment". This is when newborn babies crawl without help up the mother's stomach to find and latch onto the breast. (Dr Righard has produced a video showing this (5)). This happens best in the first hour after birth when the baby is awake and alert. If you have not had a chance to do this with your prem baby, be encouraged that it can happen even days after birth. Putting your baby in skin-to-skin contact on your chest and leaving her next to the breast will help breastfeeding to start normally. This is discussed in more detail under breastfeeding. Attachment parenting is discussed in the chapter on the long-term benefits of skin-to-skin contact. SSC babies are cuddled more even a year later.

Firm holding is what she needs now; this is called "containment". Feather-light touch or stroking will irritate her sensitive skin. Inside your womb she was held very tightly, so bend her legs up close to her body with her arms close to her chest. Keep her hands near her mouth as she has been comforting herself like this for months. It is called "self-soothing" and will help her to be more peaceful and less stressed.

If you have had a caesarean section, dad or a nurse can hold your prem on your chest. Some hospitals will encourage dad to hold her skin-to-skin contact on his chest inside his shirt. She will know his voice from the months inside you and it is a wonderful time for dad to bond with his baby and to feel that he can help as well. (A dad will also feel helpless and worried when their baby is born too early.) Remember that skin-to-skin contact means no bra for mum and no clothes on your prem except a tiny nappy and baby must be held under your shirt.

Now a wonderful thing can happen: your body will automatically warm up to warm your baby if she is cold and will cool down if your baby is hot!. Your body's biology is wonderful! Studies have shown that for twins, a mum's breasts can have different temperatures depending on what each twin needs (7). Your body will keep your baby's temperature more stable than an incubator can. (This automatic temperature change does not work as well for dads (8). There is more for dads in a later chapter.)

It is important that your prem does not get cold as she has a chemical called "surfactant" in her lungs which help her to breathe. If she gets cold, this chemical becomes more solid and she will struggle to breathe. (She may need to be given this chemical to help her lungs work properly.) All first aid courses speak of A, B and C: airway, breathing and circulation. Your baby will need the same checking as she is born. Your baby's tiny neck is not strong and her airway will need to be supported in the sniffing position to help her to breathe. As she has her first sleep she may be need to be fixed onto your chest to stabilize her airway. She may need extra oxygen and she can get this through a tube while she is on your chest.

There are many reasons for premature births and your baby may need to be taken into the NICU. Try to be with her as much as possible and hold her skin-to-skin even with all the tubes and monitors attached.

Medical staff have traditionally stabilized babies in incubators and firmly believed in this method. But all studies have shown that skin-to-skin contact stabilizes heart rate and oxygen saturation of babies better and faster than in an incubator, even very small babies of 27 weeks gestation! (If the doctors and nurses are sceptical, leave all the monitors attached and your baby's stability will speak for itself (3)).

Technical support can be added when your prem is in skin-to-skin contact. This may mean systems changes in your NICU – encourage the nurses and doctors to look at the references on the "fine print pages" (9;10).

Talk to your baby

Ask for a chair to sit next to your baby so you can hold her and talk to her. You can still hold her skin-to-skin when she has oxygen and heart monitors – this will help her to stabilize. It will also help you to feel like her mum and dad and to love her. (Parents of prems have not had all the usual months to prepare mentally for being parents, and need time to realize that they are parents to their very tiny baby.)

Your baby needs your breast milk to give her the antibodies she needs to protect her. If you can, call in a lactation consultant or breastfeeding assistant to get your breast milk started. If you do want to breastfeed, start pumping straight away. You will have more success if you start within 6 hours of birth. Keeping your baby in skin-to-skin contact with her nuzzling your chest will help to produce prolactin, the hormone which makes the milk.

Your milk will not be the same as the milk for a full term baby. Your body knows that it needs to produce breast milk that will give your prem the proteins for brain growth that she would have been getting through the umbilical cord. If she is a very tiny prem she may not yet be strong enough to suckle from your breast, but she still needs breast milk. Express it and feed it to her through a tube in her nose or mouth that goes straight into her stomach. Feed her little amounts often as her stomach is so tiny. Express your milk more often and more milk will be produced. Even if there are only two drops of the early milk, colostrum, it will be enough to help her stomach to be healthy. Colostrum is called "white gold" because of all the antibodies which it contains to protect the tiny baby from germs. She does not need formula. Formula is milk designed for a baby cow and only has about 30 nutrients; your breast milk will give her the 1200 nutrients that a human baby needs for her brain to grow properly.

Sucking from a bottle is stressful and tiring for babies as they cannot breathe and suck from a bottle at the same time (11;12). Write on her card that you insist that she is not given a bottle. Feeding her your expressed milk in a tiny cup is better for her. Remember that your aim is to get her breastfeeding as soon as possible.

Premature babies need breast milk even more than full term babies to help them to grow properly and for their brains to grow healthy. With support, prems can breastfeed at 28 weeks.

So do not let the hospital say that your prem baby cannot breastfeed until she is 32 weeks gestation or a specific weight. Ask for a lactation consultant to help you. Pay for it if you need to; it is well worth it as your baby will have far fewer illness and allergy problems later in her life.

Your prem has been born too early and the first few hours may have been spent desperately trying to keep your tiny baby alive. Now she is breathing and her heart is working and breastfeeding has started. You and your baby should continue to be one unit as you have been for months.

Now, what about you?

First, take a deep breath and be grateful!

Often, when the hours of crisis are over, the baby is more stable but you, her parents, are feeling completely exhausted. Now that your prem has settled, you may be struggling yourself.

Having a prem baby is a major life shock. Your emotions will feel upside down.

It is OK to cry; in fact tears bring healing, calmness and relief.

It has happened, and needs to be accepted. You as parents need to talk about it together and support each other.

What do you do now?

It is time to take stock and find out what YOU as parents need.

Do you need more information on how to cope emotionally? You will find a chapter on this further on.

Maybe you want to find out more about the technology or medicines that your baby needs. Knowing more can make you feel less helpless and out of control. Ask the staff "what are these wires and tubes connected to my baby?" You can also start learning about the details of the technical support that prems may need (see the technology chapter). It is worth finding out as much as you can about your baby's needs and the medicines and machines that are helping her. You will be part of the team, and not just a victim or bystander.

Have you given your baby a name? Often, parents are too scared to do this in case their baby does not survive. Your baby has been a person for months already inside you.. Give her a name, a name that you say softly to her whenever you spend time with her; her name that you say gently to comfort her. (You need to call her something as you speak to her ... perhaps you had a nickname for her while she was inside you ... maybe she even recognizes that for the time being!) Obviously this will depend on cultural and religious traditions.

Have you let your friends and family know of your baby's birth? They are more likely to support you.

FIRST DAY CHECKLIST:

Have you given your child a name? ....

Have you taken her picture? ....

(Remember not to use a flash when taking photographs as this will hurt your prem's fragile eyes.)

Your own baby's FACT SHEET

Mum's name ....

Dad's name ....

Baby's name ....

Birth date ....

Time of birth ....

Weight at birth ....

Length at birth ....

Place of birth ....

Ask the staff to write down your baby's diagnosis and medication that you want to understand better ....

....

....

Baby's questions

How did you choose my name?

....

....

....

When did you first hold me? ....

When was my first breastfeed? ....

Doctors and nurses who helped me: ....

....

....

....

Use space below for handprint and footprint!

Parents' questions about NICU

Does your hospital allow skin-to-skin contact at birth?..

Does your NICU encourage skin-to-skin contact – or insist on it?...

For full term babies?.. For prems?..

Is there a place for you, her mum or dad to sit with your baby in skin-to-skin contact?

Can parents sleep in the hospital if they have a prem baby?..

Fine Print Page - Introduction

This chapter summarises many things, and the fine print on them will be found in later chapters. For example, the statements about your baby's brain needs, and separation, will be discussed in the fine print page in the Neuroscience chapter. Just for starters, here are some annotations.

1. Without ventilators or incubators, but using mothers as incubators, survival improved from 10% to 50% in a study in Zimbabwe. Both authors were involved in developing the technique.
2. This "dying infant" went on to survive. Care should be taken not to instil false hope for such "miracles" – See Compassionate Care chapter. . However, if the baby improves, it deserves full care.
3. In this randomized controlled trial, babies were between 1200g and 2200g. Those placed SSC from birth ALL stabilized after 6 hours, but only HALF those in incubators did so. The key is no separation, and starting from birth.
4. The research on self-attachment started in Sweden, where researchers were studying how much warmth and extra sugar newborn babies needed. They found that undrugged babies that were left on their mum's chest all crawled by themselves unaided to the breast and started breastfeeding. After one hour, they had higher blood sugars than those given glucose, and they were much warmer.
5. Dr Righard has produced a video of this work, available from   www.geddesproduction.com   Dr Smillie has produced a video showing that this works days and weeks later, available same website.
6. Suctioning "seemed unpleasant" and caused retching, and delayed breastfeeding behaviour.
7. Susan Ludington has researched temperature effects on twins: "thermal synchrony" between mother and child ensures a very stable temperature, one degree higher than incubator.
8. Dads tend to increase baby's temperature, but not dangerously, as the baby self-regulates by wriggling to cooler spots or putting out an arm.
9-10. Here are detailed descriptions of techniques combining SSC and ventilation. Two of the most thorough covering many technical details are by Susan Ludington.
11-12. There is a general belief that bottle is less stressful than breast, but there is no evidence to support this. Paula Meier researched this in 32 week infants who were bottle and breastfeeding; babies had lower oxygen both during and after bottle-feeding. Mizuno studied the musculature and pressures during both, and politely notes them to be different !

Reference List

(1) Bergman NJ, Jurisoo LA. The 'kangaroo-method' for treating low birth weight babies in a developing country. Trop Doct 1994 April;24(2):57-60.
(2) Ludington-Hoe SM. Kangaroo Care The best you can do for your infant. Bantam Books; 1993.
(3) Bergman NJ, Linley LL, Fawcus SR. Randomized controlled trial of skin-to-skin contact from birth versus conventional incubator for physiological stabilization in 1200- to 2199-gram newborns. Acta Paediatr 2004 June;93(6):779-85.
(4) Christensson K, Siles C, Moreno L, Belaustequi A, de la FP, Lagercrantz H et al. Temperature, metabolic adaptation and crying in healthy full-term newborns cared for skin-to-skin or in a cot. Acta Paediatrica (Oslo, Norway: 1992) 1992 June;81(6-7):488-93.
(5) Righard L, Alade MO. Effect of delivery room routines on success of first breast-feed. Lancet 1990 November 3;336(8723):1105-7.
(6) Widstrom AM, Ransjo-Arvidson AB, Christensson K, Matthiesen AS, Winberg J, Uvnas-Moberg K. Gastric suction in healthy newborn infants. Effects on circulation and developing feeding behaviour. Acta Paediatr Scand 1987 July;76(4):566-72.
(7) Ludington-Hoe Sm, Lewis T, Morgan K, Cong X, Anderson L, Reese S. Breast-infant temperature synchrony with twins during shared kangaroo care. JOGNN 2006;35(2):1-9.
(8) Ludington-Hoe SM, Hashemi MS, Argote LA, Medellin G, Rey H. Selected physiologic measures and behavior during paternal skin contact with Colombian preterm infants. J Dev Physiol 1992 November;18(5):223-32.
(9) Ludington-Hoe Sm, Ferreira C, Swinth J, Ceccardi JJ. afe Criteria and Procedure for Kangaroo Care with intubated Preterm Infants. JOGNN 2007;32(2003):579-88.
(10) Ludington-Hoe Sm, Morgan K, Abouelfettah A. A clinical guideline for implemetation of kangaroo care with premature infants of 30 or more weeks' postmenstrual age. Advances in Neonatal Care 2008;8(3 S):S3-S23.
(11) Meier P. Bottle- and breast-feeding: effects on transcutaneous oxygen pressure and temperature in preterm infants. Nursing Research 1988 January;37(1):36-41.
(12) Mizuno K, Ueda A. Changes in Sucking Performance from Nonnutritive Sucking to Nutritive Sucking during Breast-and-Bottle-Feeding. Pediatr Res 2006;59(5):728-7.

HOW PREMS ARE DIFFERENT FROM FULL-TERM NEWBORNS

You may get a shock when you first see her as prems often look different to full term babies. She has not had time to grow in size and put on weight and be nicely rounded.

> **Be reassured; she will grow to look "normal" in time.**

She may look:

- very tiny, like a little wizened old woman with a wrinkled face.
- Her head may look too large for her body size and be longer and thinner. Her head bones are soft.
- Her body and head are big but her skinny arms may make her look like an underfed child.
- Her ribs may stick out, and may cave in with each breath.
- Her arms and legs often look too long and too thin and will often be straight out, not bent or flexed.
- Her skin is thin, fragile and shiny, and wrinkled. Her skin may change colour depending on the amount of oxygen in her blood.
- Your prem's eyes may stay closed because her eyes are so sensitive to light.
- Your prem's hands and feet are often perfectly formed, just long and thin.
- Her ears may be very soft and unformed.
- She may have hair on her body, especially the shoulders.
- She may need lots of tubes and machines to help her survive as her tiny body may not be ready to cope on her own. This is often the most scary thing for parents to see.

Inside the premature baby the body systems are immature.

- Her heart may beat very irregularly.
- Her lungs may struggle to breathe.
- Her central nervous system is immature so she may twitch more.
- Her digestive system may take time to work properly.
- Your prem's immune system is immature and will need your colostrum or first milk to help protect her.

A full-term baby would have 40 weeks inside the mother where all her needs are provided.

As a full-term baby is born, huge changes are needed for the new-born to cope in her new environment. These adjustments for heart, lungs, temperature and immune and metabolic control can be overwhelming, or life-threatening.

> **These changes are even more difficult for your prem to make.**

Prems are pre-mature babies. They are born too early and are not fully ready to make the huge adjustments to life outside the mother. The prem of 24 weeks gestation should have had another 16 weeks in her mother's womb. With improved technology and feeding, preterm babies are surviving at earlier and earlier ages. In the past, neonatal care was focused on survival. This meant support was needed for the immature body and her developing lungs and heart. Modern neonatal care is now focusing on the <u>quality</u> of survival, and how to improve the long term brain development to achieve a good future for that child.

Firstly – your tiny new baby has been born too early and so she is called a "premature" or prem. There are two measures of maturity, namely age and weight. Full gestation is regarded as 40 weeks (nine months plus one week). Any early birth from 24 weeks to 37 weeks gestation is a premature birth. Technically, babies over 37 weeks are not seen as being premature. Generally, the longer the tiny developing baby stays in her mother's womb, the better she can cope – inside mum is where her body is designed to grow best. Mostly, the more premature the baby is, the more problems she has. The gestational age is usually assessed before birth, but can also be measured by scoring certain physical features. Weight is less important, but generally the lower the weight, the more problems the prem faces. Babies can be both premature and small for their age.

Abbreviations:	**Translated**	**Meaning**
GA	Gestational Age	The weeks from conception to birth
SGA	Small for Gestational Age	A premature baby who is too small for her gestational age (because of malnutrition, mother smoking, etc.)
AGA	Appropriate for Gestational Age	A premature baby is smaller than a full term, but the right size for her gestational age
LBW	Low birth weight.	baby below 2,5kg (5.5 lbs)
VLBW	Very low birth weight	Below 1500g (3.3lbs)
ELBW	Extremely low birth weight	below 1000g (2.2lbs)

<u>Inside her mother the fetus has</u>
▸   oxygen and food that are provided through the placenta;
▸   no need to breathe or digest;
▸   a stable temperature;
▸   a safe place to curl up;

▸   constant gentle sounds – mum's heartbeat, muffled voices and other sounds;

▸   the day – night rhythms of her mum;

▸   no need to respond to lots of messages and distractions – her nervous system is protected;

▸   no lights.

Outside mother the prem is not able to regulate her own body.

Physical development:

▸   her heart rate and breathing are uneven;

▸   she changes colour often.

Motor development:

▸   she is tense, her muscles twitch and she trembles;

▸   she is likely to be stiff, but she may be limp;

▸   she can't stay curled up.

Consciousness:

▸   she can't be alert;

▸   she is fussy and unsettled;

▸   she can't focus on you for a long time;

▸   she gets tired quickly;

▸   she struggles to calm down after being disturbed.

What a difference skin-to-skin contact can make!

Mum and Dad, you can help your baby's body temperature to stay constant, and her breathing and heart rate to stabilize. You are absolutely essential for your prem's best care, so make the time now to be there for your baby. Both parents are needed so that there is less stress caused by separation.

> **What your baby looks like will depend on how many weeks premature she was born.**

She has been born early and is <u>very</u> tiny.   If she is more than 8 weeks premature she may look very different to a full term baby and may need high-tech assistance to help breathing.

As you look at her it may be a shock as she has not had time to grow in size and put on weight and be nicely rounded. Some parents say their prems look like little wizened old women. It may be a shock to see how tiny she is, but look at her perfect fingers and toes – she is "fearfully and wonderfully made".

Some parents of prems comment on the wonder of being able to watch their baby grow; if she had not been born early they would not be able to see that development.

The prem's head often looks larger than normal in relation to her body size. She loses most of her heat through her head so she may need to keep a cap on.

If a prem is in an incubator, her head may become longer and thinner, not stay rounded. Her head can also become flattened as the skull bones are still soft.

Body: her body is big and her head is big but her skinny arms may make her look like an underfed child. Her ribs often stick out and may cave in with each breath. This chest breathing is a sign of stress. She may struggle to breathe as her lungs are not ready and she may need help from a ventilator. As she grows she will change from this chest breathing to stomach breathing which is better. Even tiny prems change to this stable abdominal breathing when they have skin-to-skin contact.

Arms and legs: the arms and legs often look too long and too thin as the fat tissue has not been put in place. The arms and legs will often be straight out, not flexed.

Skin: her skin is thin, fragile and shiny. The colour depends on what is happening underneath the skin. If she has good oxygenation, then the prem is rosy and pink. Prems often look blue as they struggle to get enough oxygen. Prems don't have a layer of stored fat under their skin so the skin often looks wrinkled. It may also look wrinkled if the baby has lost fat. SGA babies may have needed to use some of their stored fat before they were born if the placenta was not working properly (for example). ELBW babies have skin that leaks water. These "aquapores" close after 1–2 days.

Hair on the body: between 28 weeks and 36 weeks of development, the human fetus often has hair on the shoulders and back. Sometimes prems have that hair too – it is called lanugo. This is normal and will disappear in time.

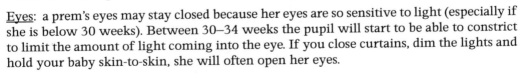

Eyes: a prem's eyes may stay closed because her eyes are so sensitive to light (especially if she is below 30 weeks). Between 30–34 weeks the pupil will start to be able to constrict to limit the amount of light coming into the eye. If you close curtains, dim the lights and hold your baby skin-to-skin, she will often open her eyes.

Hands and feet: the prem's hands and feet are often perfectly formed, just long and thin. If the baby is born before 24 weeks there are often no creases on the soles of the feet, or on the hands. Often the prem's toenails and fingernails are not yet formed. These signs help doctors to score the baby's age.

Ears: only from 28 weeks onwards does the outer ear begin to stiffen as the cartilage of the ear does not develop before then. Before 35 weeks your prem's ears may be floppy. Ear development also helps doctors score the age of the baby.

<u>Muscles</u>: prem babies often have low muscle tone and so appear "floppy".

<u>Genitalia</u>: these may be very underdeveloped in a prem and may look strange. Do not worry.

There are many reasons for prematurity. Your prem's need for specific support and technology will depend on her gestational age and stability. Each prem's needs are unique.

Parents need to know about the various organs and systems

The premature baby has <u>immature</u> body systems.

- ▶ Heart
- ▶ Lungs
- ▶ Central Nervous system
- ▶ Endocrine system
- ▶ Digestive system
- ▶ Immune system

The body is still preparing for birth so the lungs, gut and kidneys need to develop.

A baby's lungs expect to mature just before birth at 40 weeks. It is the stress of being born that helps them to mature As she has been born early, the prem's lungs are not fully developed and she may need help from machines for breathing, extra oxygen or surfactant. Steroids are often given to premature infants before birth to make the lungs mature.

You need to understand the technology that is helping your baby to survive. I will translate the technical words used in the NICU in a later chapter.

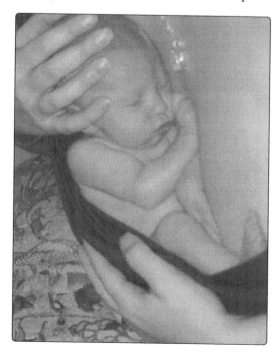

Your baby's birthweight ....

Her gestation ....

Mark an "X" on the gestation age scale for your own baby.
Then mark an "X" for the birth weight of your own baby.
Now draw an arrow from the top "X" to the bottom "X"

GESTATION Age (weeks)	24w	26w	28w	30w	32w	34w	36w	38w	40w

WEIGHT at birth	800g	900g	1100g	1300g	1700g	2000g	2600g	2900g	3200g

If the arrow points straight down, then your baby is normal, or usual, weight for that womb age.
If the arrow leans a little bit in either direction, it is also probably normal.
If the arrow leans more backwards, (down to the left), then your baby is small for its gestation
If the arrow leans forward (down to the right), then your baby is large for its gestation.

WHAT PARENTS CAN DO TO HELP THEIR BABY

Mum and Dad, you can both do a lot for your baby.

The most important things are to:

> ▶ BE THERE WITH HER
> ▶ HOLD YOUR PREM
> ▶ GET INVOLVED IN HER CARE

Mum's chest provides the place for the smoothest changeover from life in the womb to life in the world. It is the safe place where all of your baby's needs can be met. Mum provides emotional **continuity** of love, security and relationship so that her baby does not become stressed.

> **A baby is more stable on her mother's chest than in an incubator. The more premature the baby is, the more she needs her mother to reach stability.**

Even a 28 week prem can breathe properly on her mother's chest, can breastfeed properly, and all her body systems can adapt better to her new life.

<u>Dads have a vital role to play</u>:

You can hold your baby skin-to-skin, especially if Mum has had a Caesarean section.

You can feed her through a tube or cup-feed her the breast milk.

You can change nappies, bath her, etc.

The only thing dad can't do is breastfeed! ☺

Skin-to-skin contact and breastfeeding provide stability for the newborn. The mother's body provides the continuity of sensations that the baby's brain needs, and the baby's brain in turn controls the body of the baby.

On parent's chest	Incubator: (separated)
Unstressed baby	Stressed baby
Respiratory Rate more even	Breathing often irregular
Heart rate normal	HR faster
Temperature slightly higher than incubator and in a very small range	Big fluctuations in temperature
Self attachment and bonding	Protest crying
Breastfeeding and growth	Dissociation and survival but little growth
Breast milk provides immune protection and nutritional needs	No immune protection at all from cows milk, and only about 10%nutritional needs are provided
Best sensory stimulation so the baby has emotional well-being	Harmful stimuli to the brain
Absorbs food in the gut well	Gut absorption has shut down
Grows faster (30g/day)	Grows slower (10g/day)

This section is addressed to fathers, but I know that in some situations fathers may be absent or not willing to be part of this process. This may bring up its own set of issues and emotions to deal with. As I have said above, get help! The broader family and friends can be a wonderful support.

Dad: you have a vital role to play in the life of your premature infant!

<u>How a dad can help his baby:</u>

Nothing can properly prepare you for the time of watching your tiny baby struggling to breathe or lying on her back with tubes and lines and monitors all over her tiny body. But if you hold her on your chest you experience being her father! You can do so much for her! Your baby will recognize your voice from all those months inside mum. Talk to her if she is in an incubator, and you can also carry her skin-to-skin. Sometimes Dad can hold his baby while Mum recovers from a caesarean section. This can be a wonderful and beautiful time as you bond with your tiny baby. Your baby needs you – and so does the mother of your baby.

You may be shocked at her premature birth and feel absolutely helpless. It is normal and OK to feel like this. It is normal to go through a whole range of scary emotions. I will explain these later in the workbook. What is very important is that you allow yourself to feel these emotions and express them. Do not try to deny what you are feeling. It can be very frustrating not being in control of the situation, especially if you feel that you have to take responsibility for your family. You may feel angry or helpless. You need to be involved, find out as much as possible about your prem and her medications. Ask for professional help if you are not coping.

You can share in providing all your baby's care. There are only two things you cannot do; you can't breastfeed and your temperature may not adjust as the mother's does when you hold your prem in skin-to-skin contact (1). Dads tend to overheat their babies, but that is usually not a problem as your baby will stick out an arm to cool herself down. If you are holding your baby, do not put a cap on her. Otherwise, you can do everything just as well as mum (2;3).

If your wife is expressing milk, you can feed your baby with this milk through the naso-gastric tube with a syringe, or cup feed her. You can hold her; read to her; sleep with her on your chest; help with nesting and positioning. You can also help to find out information on the websites. You can find out all about the machines and medications your baby needs. You can also read her charts and ask staff members to explain them and tell you how your baby is doing whenever you come in to be with her.

You also can have a wonderfully supportive role to play in challenging the doctors and nurses, asking for developmental care, being a champion for your baby to get the very best care possible for her.

Helping baby's mum:

You can help your wife by reading this book and discussing each chapter!

When you get involved, Mum will be relieved and feel that you are lifting her load.

Share your feelings with your wife or partner and share the experience. It is a difficult time for any relationship and you will need to keep communicating. It can be hard to be apart if Mum stays in hospital but try to find times when you can be together. Your wife or partner may be emotionally upside-down because of hormones or extreme stress. BE there for her and share it with her. One important thing that you can do is to reassure her. She may feel that your baby being born too early is her "fault". It is not. Support her and do not blame her.

Dad, if you have other small children at home just being at home with them may be the most wonderful support you can give.

Sometimes you can hold your prem baby in skin-to-skin contact (kangaroo care) while her mother goes home to rest or to give attention to another child.

In many parts of the world, dads are doing a lot of the skin-to-skin contact (SSC). In Sweden, where there is a strong social security system and dads are given a lot of paternity leave, dads and mums often share the 24 hours of skin-to-skin contact between them. It is also almost routine for Dad to hold his baby in SSC after caesarean section (4). These dads have reported that the time each spent with his prem in skin-to-skin contact in the NICU has formed a very special bond with his baby which will be the basis of a trusting relationship all her life.

Find ways of helping with the simple, practical care of your baby, including giving feeds before baby is able to breastfeed (5). Often, a dad is able to react more practically in the time soon after a prem birth, and so developing this new relationship with your child can start earlier (6;7).

What of the above would be your next step to help your prem?

....

....

....

....

....

And after that, what will you do?

....

....

....

....

....

....

....

Benefits of skin-to-skin contact for dads!

- ▶ You are empowered to care for your baby and do not feel helpless or useless,
- ▶ You are central to the caring team,
- ▶ Better bonding,
- ▶ Emotional healing,
- ▶ You are calmer and more relaxed,
- ▶ You are able to read your baby's unique cues for hunger or stress,
- ▶ You can get more sleep.

This section has covered the unexpected premature birth, and the next chapter looks at the rollercoaster of emotions that you may go through. Your baby is dependent on you to be involved early on, and to work through these issues with the support of your family.

> **Write down some of your own thoughts or experiences in the space below if you wish. You may never have done this kind of thing before. Try it! If you are used to doing this, buy a diary. You may not remember this time in NICU in future, but may find this record valuable. Maybe you will even share it with your child when she is an adult!**

....

....

....

....

....

....

....

....

....

....

....

....

....

....

....

Are you artistic? What about making a sketch of your baby?

Take photos of her but remember not to use the flash as the bright light will hurt her sensitive eyes.

Fine Print Page

This page is only about Dads, the evidence in the summary on Mums will come in other chapters. There is surprisingly little research done on dads during the period before and after birth, and even less on dads doing skin-to-skin contact.

1. Susan Ludington has been mentioned already, in her study fathers warmed their babies too well!
2. German researchers have studied babies between 28 and 31 weeks, just 11 babies, but measured in detail. They concluded there was no real difference on mum or dad in oxygen consumption, carbon dioxide production, energy expenditure, skin and rectal temperatures, heart and respiratory rates, arterial saturation, and behavioral states. They found "no adverse effects", and from reports both parents provide long periods of SSC to their prems in most German NICU's.
3. The Swedish researchers mentioned earlier studied babies after caesarean section managed in cot compared to father's skin. They reported that the blood glucose levels while on fathers skin in the first 2 hours actually increased … and it could not have been due to breastfeeding !! The temperatures were also higher than when cared for in a cot or an incubator, and surprisingly they were higher even 24 hours later.
4. This paper describes greatly reduced infant crying while on father's skin, with infants falling asleep after one hour.
5. Being involved practically, in this paper with feeding specifically, was an important element in paternal-infant bonding.
6. Mothers and fathers were interviewed about their reactions to premature birth. Both were taken by surprise, but fathers were more "ready to be involved immediately". For mothers the prem birth meant a "temporarily lost relationship", but for fathers this was new relationship just starting.
7. A hand book for fathers – not just for dads of prematures

Reference List

(1) Ludington-Hoe SM, Hashemi MS, Argote LA, Medellin G, Rey H. Selected physiologic measures and behavior during paternal skin contact with Colombian preterm infants. J Dev Physiol 1992 November;18(5):223-32.
(2) Bauer J, Sontheimer D, Fischer C, Linderkamp O. Metabolic rate and energy balance in very low birth weight infants during kangaroo holding by their mothers and fathers. J Pediatr 1996 October;129(4):608-11.
(3) Christensson K. Fathers can effectively achieve heat conservation in healthy newborn infants. Acta Paediatr 1996 November;85(11):1354-60.
(4) Erlandsson K, Dsilna A, Fagerberg I, Christensson K. Skin-to-Skin Care with the Father after Cesarean Birth and Its Effect on Newborn Crying and Prefeeding Behavior. Birth: Issues in Perinatal Care 2007 June;34(2):105-14.
(5) Taubenheim AM. Paternal--infant bonding in the first-time father. JOGN Nursing; Journal Of Obstetric, Gynecologic, And Neonatal Nursing 1981 July;10(4):261-4.
(6) Fegran L, Helseth S, Fagermoen MS. A comparison of mothers' and fathers' experiences of the attachment process in a neonatal intensive care unit. Journal of Clinical Nursing 2008 March 15;17(6):810-6.
(7) Houser PM. Fathers-To-Be Handbook: A road map for the transition to fatherhood. 1st ed. South Portland, Maine 04106: Creative Life Systems; 2009.

EMOTIONS AND COPING

Nothing can fully prepare you for parenting a prem.

You have to learn on the job.

There are many things you can do, but the key things are
- Get involved in caring for your baby.
- Talk to other parents, talk to counsellors, a social worker or a nurse
- CRY
- Ask for support and help if it feels like too much.

You may be overwhelmed by having a prem baby. It may be very scary for you worrying if your baby will survive. It is normal and OK to have these upside-down feelings and emotions. As parents you may both be under huge strain and worry. Try to keep sharing your feelings and supporting each other. It is also important to face the feelings and work through them so that you can help your baby.

Ask for help if you are struggling.

Your child needs a name!!

Some parents do not want to name their child, because they do not want to bond with her in case she dies. <u>But</u> your baby desperately <u>needs</u> you to bond with her and needs your love, your prayers, your longing for her, to help her to survive.

Many parents of prems have not had the last few weeks of pregnancy to finalise the choice of a name but it is very important.

Mothers and fathers usually have 9 months of pregnancy to prepare themselves mentally and emotionally for their new baby. When their baby is born early they are not ready or prepared. If it has been a high risk pregnancy or there is more than one baby, parents may have had some time to prepare, but that is also very stressful. There may have been problems with Mum's health and she may already have spent days or weeks in hospital.

At the onset of preterm labour, there is often a lot of anxiety and fear. Your dream of having the suitcases packed and the baby's room decorated ready to receive her is shattered as you drive to the hospital. Something is wrong and your baby is being born prematurely. As this is often a time when doctors and nurses are desperately working to keep your baby alive, they may not have time to give you all the information you need. The first view of your tiny baby may be very scary. She looks so very small and frail, and not at all like the full-term baby that you were expecting. She may be wrinkled, have hair on her shoulders, tubes in her nose and be attached to all sorts of machines that you haven't yet learnt about. She may be struggling to breathe, and be silent, or have a very weak cry. This image of her burns its way into your mind. Somehow you need to face the reality that this tiny prem baby is your child. It is normal to wish that it was different, but try to bring your mind back to the present. You need to accept the situation <u>as it is</u> <u>and do all you can</u> to make the best of it.

<u>Have you given your child a name?</u>
This is very important in terms of coping emotionally.

It is also very scary when you wonder if your child will survive. Some parents do not want to name their child, because they do not want to bond with her in case she dies. This is inside-out thinking – your baby desperately needs you to bond with her. She needs your love, your prayers, your longing for her to help her to survive. She needs to know she is wanted to help her frail and tiny body to fight for life.

Your baby has been born too early and too small – it is a confusing, frightening time and there is always the big question –

Will my baby survive?

This manual is intended to help you navigate through the scary and confusing weeks while your child is in the NICU and to help you so that you can help your baby.

Every family is unique, each prem has her own, sometimes complex problems, and is slightly different from other prems, Your uncertainty of the future can be increased by not understanding the medical jargon. There may also be a lot of stress around the time of discharge from the hospital – "will I cope on my own?" In the case of bereavement it is even harder to bear. (This will be covered in a separate section.)

Your emotions will swing and be unstable; partly because mums body's hormones are changing, but also because this is a major life shock. You will probably go through some or all of the following emotions, not necessarily in this order, and some many times over (1)!

At this time, you may feel

▶ Overwhelming shock

▶ Disbelief or denial

▶ Grief

▶ Anticipatory grief

▶ Fear

▶ Guilt

▶ A sense of failure

▶ Anger

▶ Confusion

▶ Depressed and cry a lot

▶ Immense strain

▶ Upset with nurses

You may also find it

▶ Difficult to concentrate

▶ Difficult to sleep

Here are some of the details

You may feel overwhelming shock at the early birth.

Disbelief or denial is often a defence mechanism to stop you from attaching to an infant that may not survive.

Grief is not just grief when someone dies; in the case of a prem baby the mother and father may go through what is called "anticipatory grief", which is looking at the possibility of death of their tiny baby. As parents you may fear that she won't survive, so you may be reluctant to bond with her. Yet she desperately needs you to bond with her and love her to help her pull through. Parents may also grieve the loss of a successful pregnancy, and the loss of a dream or expectation of a healthy full-term baby. (2)

Linked to this, mum (specifically) may feel guilty, or feel that she is a failure. She may blame herself for having done something wrong, or not being "a good enough mother" to deliver a "normal" baby. Most of this feeling is false guilt. Some mums – after reading this – may feel guilty that they did not care for their prems in the best way. It is never too late to give your baby extra love! Self-doubt drains a lot of energy and is not helpful. Often this can be solved by simply asking the doctors if there was a medical reason why your baby was born prem.

Sometimes your behaviour or lifestyle could have contributed to the prematurity of your baby. Smoking and drug abuse are examples. It is best to admit such things, and resolve to put them right. Don't pretend. Rather ask for help. Work through it, deal with it and leave it behind.

You may be very tired – the delivery is still hard work, and worry also drains your energy. You may worry that your baby won't survive, or won't grow up normally.

You may be angry at your situation: "Why me?", "Why is my baby born prem?" This anger might come out as blaming your partner, or the nurses, or everybody. You may be irritable with your family when they are trying to help.

You may feel <u>very confused</u> by these strong feelings. It is especially important to remember that you have gone through a physical, hormonal and emotional roller-coaster. It takes time to find your balance. <u>Feeling depressed</u> and <u>crying</u> is very common. There is nothing wrong with crying. Tears are deeply healing and release oxytocin, which will calm you.

Some people may use the coping mechanism of being <u>over-optimistic</u>, by <u>denying the reality</u> that there is anything wrong. Be careful of this, as your partner may be in a very different space emotionally. You may find it <u>difficult to concentrate</u> on basic things; you may find it difficult to sleep because you are worrying about your baby's survival. Try to get as much rest as you can.

A premature birth can cause immense strain on any relationship. Keep talking to each other, with mutual respect and support. Try to understand each other's ways of coping. Sometimes dad has to go back to work and can only come to the hospital occasionally. Mum may feel neglected and that he does not care about the baby. Sometimes dad has taken the baby to the NICU, and has had time to learn about the machines and bond with his baby, and then mum feels left out. You may feel upset with the nurses because they are caring for your baby, not you, her mother. You may feel left out. But remember: you are special to your baby, and you are the most important medicine she can get, because only you can give her an emotionally stable environment.

One of the hardest things to cope with is <u>disappointed expectations</u>. This is particularly relevant in modern society where we believe we "should" have control over so many things, health included.

> **Every child's life is a gift to receive, not a right to demand.**

<u>What can you do to deal with these emotions</u>?

- ▶ Get involved in caring for your baby (3; 4).
- ▶ Learn her own unique behavioural cues, the things that make her stressed or relaxed.
- ▶ Give her as much skin-to-skin care as you can (5–7).
- ▶ Find out as much as you can about your baby's condition (we are often afraid of what we don't know).
- ▶ Ask questions in the NICU.
- ▶ Ask for help from family.
- ▶ Talk to other parents of prems in the NICU; they have been in your situation and are often a wonderful support and encouragement.
- ▶ Talk to a counsellor, a social worker or a nurse.
- ▶ Talk to a caring person. (It is important for dads to do that too.)
- ▶ Ask for support from Lactation Consultants, etc.
- ▶ It may be helpful to make notes of your feelings.
- ▶ Learn the names of your baby's nurses and doctors. Work with them – they are doing all the care and tests <u>for</u> your baby, not <u>to</u> her to help your baby survive.
- ▶ Allow yourself to cry.
- ▶ Your faith may be tested, but can also be a lifeline.

> ### Hope is what keeps parents going.

There is a lot you <u>can</u> do to help your tiny new baby even though you may feel helpless because she is so small and frail and fragile and may be linked to so many monitors and machines.

The weeks in NICU may be a roller coaster ride of emotion. Face those feelings.

It may be helpful to make notes of your feelings as this can help you see them more objectively. These strong emotions and worry about your baby's survival can put immense strain on any loving marriage or relationship. If you are carrying these feelings alone as a single mum or without the loving support of family members it can be very scary and lonely indeed. Worrying whether you have enough money to pay for her care is also difficult. Ask for help!

If your relationship is already strained, the shock of having a premature infant can cause immense tension between you. However, this can also be a time to work together and draw closer. Keep talking about your feelings to each other, and try to hear each other's emotions without reacting too quickly out of your own pain. Be together. Take time off for a meal or a film together.

Ideas to help Mum and Dad cope

Your baby may be in the NICU for a long time. You may need to pace yourself for the long haul, so you need to look after yourself.

- Get enough sleep. Sleep when your baby sleeps. If necessary, put up a "do not disturb" sign when you are doing skin-to-skin care.
- Eat well. You need to eat healthy snacks to keep up your immune system. If you get sick, you may not be allowed to visit or hold your baby.
- Get comfortable clothes which button down the front in soft cotton fabrics which will not hurt your baby's skin.
- Have a long bath to relax sometimes.
- Get outside each day.
- Getting exercise will help you keep life in perspective or balance.
- Have family time to be in the NICU together sometimes, not just in shifts.
- Ask for help from friends and family to look after other children.

After a week

- Have you taken a tiny footprint and handprint of your baby?
- Have you taken a weekly picture of your baby? (Do not use a flash which will damage the baby's eyes, rather use a digital camera on a tripod) and watch how quickly she grows.

- Make a tape recording of your voice to leave with your child. Your voice will soothe your baby when nothing else can.
- Keep a list of all the specialists that care for your baby. Ask for a primary nurse and doctor. Ask who is the one who makes the decisions about your baby's care.

▶ Write down important dates and file information.

▶ Read your baby's chart and ask the staff to explain (write the jargon into the section for this).

▶ Keep a journal for your thoughts. It can be very helpful to write down your thoughts through the time your baby is in the NICU. Many things will be forgotten, but often writing down the hard thoughts and stages, helps one to see the feelings more objectively. So maybe get a small notebook to keep a record of your feelings. You can also write down questions that you want to ask the doctor when you come in and write down his answers.

▶ Put up photos of your baby.

▶ Write down your baby's unique likes and dislikes on her care plan.

Below is a worksheet to help you, Mum and Dad, to identify the feelings you may experience, but not be able to describe. You may need someone to help you do so. Mum and Dad, you have work to do to look after your tiny premature baby and so you need to get to grips with yourselves and your situation as soon as possible in order to help your premature baby effectively.

COMMONLY EXPERIENCED EMOTIONS

Term	Identify	Comment	Reason to face issue
Guilt	"What did I do wrong?" "I failed as a mother." "I shouldn't have…"	This is the most common emotion.	You blame yourself so you feel paralysed.
Inadequacy	"I feel useless here." "I'm redundant, not needed."	This is a totally new situation and you have no clue what to do.	You feel paralysed.
Incompetence	"What if I do the wrong things?"	You feel disempowered	You do not want to learn the technology.
Helplessness	"I can't do anything for my baby."	You sit blankly.	You feel disempowered.
Denial	"This is not true." "This can't be happening to me." "I don't want this baby."	You have a problem with accepting your baby and your situation. This is often your mind's way of buffering or cushioning the initial shock.	Maybe you do not even want to see your baby in the NICU.

Anger	"Why me?" "My baby was whisked away." "Where has my perfect pregnancy gone?"	You feel angry at everything. "Why?" "This is **your** fault!"	Blaming others or yourself does not help anyone. You may be angry at your **baby** for messing up your life and marriage.
Bargaining	"If you save my baby, then I will …."	You may do this with your spouse or with God.	This is an unrealistic approach.
Depression	"I can't cope any more." "This is hopeless."	When you can no longer deny the reality, the anger may turn inwards to become depression.	Lots of withdrawing or crying can increase the emotional distance between you and your partner and between you and your baby.
Disappointment	"I wanted something else (perfect baby)."		
Acceptance	"It's going OK."	You have come to terms with your baby's premature birth. Your emotions will have settled.	You are able to keep going through the weeks your baby is in the NICU – this book will give you practical ways to help your baby develop.
Purpose	"We're learning a lot." "I have bonded with my baby."		There is a lot you can do practically to help your tiny new baby.

A small note on depression

You may want to withdraw and cry a lot. Do this! Tears are immensely healing and release oxytocin (feel-good hormone), which will make you feel better. It will also help mum to produce breast milk. Exhaustion from not having enough sleep because you are worrying about your premature baby in the NICU can lead to sadness or depression. Here we are looking at mood and emotion, not the clinical condition that needs to be treated with medication. (8)

"Postnatal depression" (PND) might occur separately. Ask for a professional assessment if the depression goes on for a long time. If you have struggled with depression before, or have a history of depression, it may resurface at this time of worrying about your premature baby. There are simple surveys that you can do to see if you are at risk for PND. The hospital staff would need to refer you to a local clinic for evaluation. Social workers may want to have a family meeting to try to identify support structures in the home and family and friends that can help the mum and new baby.

Do send your thoughts and experiences for the next edition of this book! This will help another set of parents in this situation!

Send to jill@kangaroomothercare.com

Write what emotions you have struggled with. If it is helpful, keep a daily diary or journal of your feelings. Sometimes seeing them on paper helps you cope better and not feel so overwhelmed.

....

....

....

....

....

....

....

....

....

....

....

....

....

....

....

....

....

....

....

....

....

....

....

....

....

HARD QUESTIONS

Parents of premature babies often have to ask hard questions. Some of these questions do not have easy or immediate answers. It is a very worrying time for parents. It is also worrying for the nurses and doctors who are fighting for your baby's life. You will need to work together and talk through these questions (9).

<u>Some of the early questions:</u>
- What are the chances that my baby will survive?
- How premature is she?
- Why was she born early?
- Whose "fault" is it?
- Is it better if she does not survive?
- What problems does she have now?
- What treatment is she getting?
- How can I help my baby in the NICU?
- Can I hold her, feed her, etc?
- How long does she have to stay in the NICU?
- How am I going to cope?
- Will I have enough money to pay for the NICU?

<u>Questions for the longer term</u>
- How will this affect the other siblings and the family?
- Will she be able to walk?
- Will she be disabled?
- Will she need special care later?
- Will she develop properly?
- Will she be able to attend a normal school?

What questions did you have?

....

....

....

....

....

....

....

....

What answers did you receive?

....

....

....

....

....

....

....

....

What are the chances that my baby will survive? (This is always the biggest question that parents of prems face.)

There are no easy answers to this and everything will depend on your baby.

Some important factors

▶   How many weeks premature was she born? (What is her gestational age?)

▶   What was her birth weight?

▶   Does she have breathing problems?

▶   Does she have birth defects/malformations?

▶   Does she have a disease or infection?

Usually the gestational age is the most important because it will decide if her body organs, particularly her lungs, are developed enough.

Ask your doctor for honest answers. Some babies suddenly get sick and die, others are tiny fighters and keep going even though they have lots of problems.

Survival for high-tech NICUs for the USA and Europe:

▶   Less than 21 weeks – no babies will survive

▶   22 weeks – Very few survive

▶   23 weeks   5 – 25%

▶   24 weeks   40 – 60% *   sudden big jump

▶   25 weeks   50 – 80%

▶   26 weeks   80 – 90%

▶   27 weeks   over 90%

* There is a big jump at 24 weeks of gestational age because the lungs are more mature at this point. From 28 weeks, survival in modern NICUs is very good.

See the end of this workbook for the different types of support that are available in terms of networks, organizations, people, internet sites and books.

Fine Print Page – Emotions and Coping

1. Bakewell et al provide a framework for comprehensive care that includes specifically aspects related to emotional support to parents.
2. This review identifies and examines common content and processes of postpartum counseling interventions to address trauma symptoms following childbirth. It identifies many of these emotions, while concluding that evidence on how to manage them is lacking!
3. In the past, NICU's discouraged parents from visiting … they and their infants suffered! Parental involvement is essential for subsequent quality outcome.
4. As parents engage, their competence increases, and their contribution to care likewise. They become empowered.
5. Skin-to-skin contact is not the focus of this chapter, but SSC does have profound effects on parent's moods, emotions and empowerment.
6. The more parents are involved, and the more SSC they give, the better the bonding and the subsequent developmental outcomes.
7. Tessier elaborates this in a "bonding hypothesis: (KMC) creates a climate in the family whereby parents become sensitive care givers. The general hypothesis is that skin-to-skin contact in the KMC group will build up a positive perception in the mothers and a state of readiness to detect and respond to infant's cues."
8. Depression is common and easily overlooked. SSC may directly improve this.
9. This article looks at maternal emotions to low birth weight infants. Quote: "It is possible that among mothers of VLBW infants, for whom none of the oxytocin-releasing conditions were met, oxytocin never reached the level required to activate the development of maternal behavior. Intervention efforts that aim to enhance proximity and touch in VLBW infants, such as skin-to-skin contact , may be crucial for these mothers in order to initiate the bonding process."

Reference List

(1) Bakewell-Sachs S, Gennaro S. Parenting the post-NICU premature infant. MCN The American Journal Of Maternal Child Nursing 2004 November;29(6):398-403.
(2) Gamble J, Creedy D. Content and Processes of Postpartum Counseling After a Distressing Birth Experience: A Review. Birth: Issues in Perinatal Care 2004 September;31(3):213-8.
(3) Latva R, Lehtonen L, Salmelin RK, Tamminen T. Visiting less than every day: a marker for later behavioral problems in Finnish preterm infants. Archives Of Pediatrics & Adolescent Medicine 2004 December;158(12):1153-7.
(4) Levy-Shiff R, Sharir H, Mogilner BM. Mother and father preterm infant relationship in the preterm nursery. Child Dev 1989;60(1):93-102.
(5) de Macedo EC, Cruvinel F, Lukasova K, D'Antino ME. The mood variation in mothers of preterm infants in Kangaroo mother care and conventional incubator care. J Trop Pediatr 2007 October 19;53(5):344-6.
(6) Feldman R. Mother-Infant Skin-to-Skin Contact (Kangaroo Care). Infants & Young Children: An Interdisciplinary Journal of Special Care Practices 2004 April;17(2):145-61.
(7) Tessier R, Cristo M, Velez S, Giron M, de Calume ZF, Ruiz-Palaez JG et al. Kangaroo mother care and the bonding hypothesis. Pediatrics 1998 August;102(2):e17 & 390-391.
(8) Dombrowski MA, Anderson GC, Santori C, Burkhammer M. Kangaroo (skin-to-skin) care with a postpartum woman who felt depressed. MCN The American Journal Of Maternal Child Nursing 2001 July;26(4):214-6.
(9) Feldman R, Weller A, Leckman JF, Kuint J, Eidelman AI. The nature of the mother's tie to her infant: maternal bonding under conditions of proximity, separation, and potential loss. Journal Of Child Psychology And Psychiatry, And Allied Disciplines 1999 September;40(6):929-39.

SKIN-TO-SKIN CONTACT

Any mother or father who has sat watching their little prem in an incubator struggling to breathe knows that feeling of utter helplessness and despair, and the agony of leaving their tiny baby so alone in hospital. But there is an alternative! It is "skin-to-skin contact".

HOLD YOUR PREM!

What is skin-to-skin contact?

- Put your naked baby onto your bare chest
- She can have on a tiny nappy and a cap if it is very cold
- Your body will keep her warm
- Your arms will support her and make her feel loved
- Cover her with a folded cloth or your shirt.
- She feels SAFE with you so her heart rate, blood pressure and oxygen amounts stabilise
- Emotionally she feels SAFE too
- She may smell her way to Mums nipple and start to breastfeed

You have replaced the incubator with your love and care and warmth

> **Skin-to-skin contact should be given to every full term baby at birth.**
> **It is even more important for fragile premature babies to help them stabilise sooner (4).**

When tied on safely in skin-to-skin contact with her airway protected, your baby can sleep on your chest as you sleep or walk around.

You can do skin-to-skin contact with a baby on a ventilator or other machines (5).

Your baby will feel SAFE with the familiar sound of your heartbeat, and voice, your warmth and your smell. This feeling of being SAFE helps the baby's heart rate to become even, stable or "regulated." Her blood pressure will be more steady and she will be able to get oxygen around her body properly. As she will feel calmed by your body her stomach can absorb your breast milk so she will grow well and healthy. Your body helps stabilise or regulate your baby's body, so she will sooner be able to regulate herself. If she has stress, she can come back to a stable point more quickly.

Her emotions will also be healthy as she feels held, secure, loved and protected so she will bond with you.

Your chest becomes the natural place of growth; she was inside you, but now can "continue the pregnancy" on your chest. Your body provides her with the warmth, protection and food that she needs for growth and the security that she needs to wire her brain for healthy relationships.

Skin-to-skin contact is close, direct skin contact between you and your prem. You can be with her for part or all of the day. Your chest becomes the natural place of growth, as a continuation of the pregnancy.

You (Mum and Dad) become your child's primary care-givers. The people working in the NICU are there to back you up and support you. You provide warmth, stability, protection. You are forming bonds with your baby which will be the emotional base of security for the rest of her life. We now know that infant mental health leads to adult mental health

You are helping your prem to stabilize and her brain to grow best just by being who you are – her mother or her father (the best people to care for her). When you put your tiny baby on your chest, her skin against your skin, she has the right smells, sounds, voice, protection, comfort (she may still need the machines for her stability).

Besides helping her to stabilize and her brain to grow, the time spent holding your baby is deeply healing for you and your little prem.

Why carry your baby skin-to-skin?

(Here is the summary, full details follow in this chapter)

Benefits of skin-to-skin contact for babies

- Better brain development
- Better emotional development
- Less stress
- Less crying
- Less brain bleeds
- More settled sleep
- Babies are more alert when they are awake
- Babies feel less pain from injections
- The heart rate stabilizes
- The oxygen saturation is more stable
- Fewer apnoea attacks
- Better breathing
- The temperature is most stable on the mother
- Breastfeeding starts more easily
- More breast milk is produced
- Gestation-specific milk is produced.
- Faster weight gain
- Baby can usually go home earlier

Benefits of skin-to-skin contact for parents

- Parents become central to the caring team
- Better bonding and interaction with their child
- Emotional healing
- Less guilt
- Parents are calmer
- Parents are empowered and more confident
- Parents are able to learn their baby's unique cues for hunger
- Parents and baby get more sleep
- Parents (especially mothers), are less depressed
- Cope better in NICU
- See baby as less "abnormal"

How to do skin-to-skin contact when your baby is born

Your baby needs only a tiny nappy and a cap.

Wash your hands well <u>every</u> time you come to your baby. Use plain soap without any perfumes.

Mum, take off your bra but keep your shirt on; it is easiest if you have one that buttons down the front. Put your baby inside your shirt, against your skin.

Sit in a chair with cushions so you can lean back and be comfortable. It is best for your baby if you are half lying, half sitting. A 30-40 degree angle helps her breathing. Place your baby on your chest facing you with her legs curled up in the foetal position. This is best for her hips. Put her tiny hands near her face for self-soothing. She has been doing that for months in the womb! You can hold your hands underneath and behind her.

Cover yourself and your prem. Your body will automatically warm up if your baby is cold, or will cool down if your baby is hot. You might find that you start to sweat; don't worry, that is normal.

If it is cold in the room, you may want to put a small cap on her head, as most of the body heat is lost through the head. For a tiny baby, losing heat means that she loses lots of calories that she should be using to grow. Make sure that all materials are pure cotton as her skin is extremely sensitive.

You may cry with relief as you hold her – that is normal. You will feel full of wonder to be able to hold your tiny baby, knowing that you are giving her the best, just by being her mother or her father. Tears are deeply healing. Mum, you will release oxytocin which will make you calmer and therefore your baby calmer too. Your tears will also help your milk production. Dad, you can cry too. You will often feel fearful as your tiny prem seems so very fragile.

Sit there for at least an hour; sleep, read a book or just enjoy your baby.

Your baby can be held in skin-to-skin contact as long as you want, for part or all of 24 hours a day. To get the full benefits of SSC, it is important for your baby to go through at least a full sleep-wake cycle which is usually about 60 minutes to get her biological systems stabilised. A tiny prem's body systems will not be mature enough for her to stabilise herself, and mother's chest will help her to settle in to a sleep-cycling and feeding rhythm.

You give closeness and security to your child. Positive feelings for your child strengthen as you care for your baby and closeness helps you to interpret your baby's unique small signals. For example, you will know very quickly when she is ready to breastfeed, is tired or stressed.

Being held skin-to-skin, contained and secure is the best thing for your prem's physical, brain and emotional health.

Note: For the first hour after birth, your baby's biology wants to be free to crawl to your breast so she can be loose (1). After the first hour, and if you want to sleep, her airway needs to be secured.

For the first six hours in skin-to-skin contact, your prem is stabilising her heart and lungs. During this time it is best to stay sitting or lying down, leaning at an angle (30-40 degrees).

Your prem baby does not have neck control; you want to prevent "obstructive apnoea" – a closed airway stopping her breathing, so it is important to secure her head firmly. To do this, place her on your chest as above. Her head should be turned to the side and tilted slightly up (sniffing position), so that her airway is protected. Take a fine weave cotton wrap and fold it under her chin and ear and around your back so she is tied firmly over your chest bone (2).

A KangaCarrier or Thari wrap can also be used. Importantly, they must not be made with stretch material as this will not keep the airways open.

Walking around

When your prem is stable enough, it may be more comfortable for you to get up and move around holding her in skin-to-skin contact (the Kangaroo Mother Care position). The wraps mentioned above make this possible.

A thari wrap

If monitors are connected to her, keep them on while you stand up the first time to confirm her stability. If she is connected to machines, you can only move as far as the leads allow.

Soon, you will be able to get up and move around more freely with your baby tied to your chest. You can read or write, talk to friends and even make tea or a meal.

Sleep

You can sleep with your prem in skin-to-skin, as long as her airway is stabilized and she is held safely in the wrap. You can lie on your back or on your side with your head slightly raised. Your baby is used to being held tightly in the womb and feels safer when she is contained. If you want to sleep with her next to you in the bed, she should have her own small bed or nest. The doctor will decide if your prem needs technical monitoring while she is sleeping.

A baby in quiet sleep should never be disturbed

When your prem starts to wake up or wriggle, you can loosen the tie and feed her. Change her nappy and spend time looking at her and talking to her.

The KangaCarrier helps you to do skin-to-skin <u>all</u> the time

Place baby in skin-to-skin contact on mother's chest bone, hands near her mouth, arms bent, legs bent (flexed).

Tie baby on tightly under chin and ear with white cloth, to fix airway.

Mother puts on KangaCarrier shirt, the first wraparound should fit tightly under baby's bottom, and include the legs.

Put second wraparound as overlap and tie firmly.

Baby is fully contained and feels safe, mother can use both hands and walk around freely.

Baby can sleep comfortably.

Mother can also sleep with baby safe.

Mother can go home 'wearing' her prem.

When she is awake, the nurses can do the tests they need to do. After that, tie her on firmly again so that she can sleep.

> **Remember that it is important for your baby to go through at least a full sleep-wake cycle which is usually about 60-90 minutes to get the full benefits of skin-to-skin contact and for brainwiring (3).**

Mum and Dad, you can take it in turns to hold your child in skin-to-skin contact. If you have twins, Dad, granny, aunt, etc can carry one twin skin-to-skin while Mum holds the other. For best effects before breastfeeding it would need to be Mum who holds the baby. If you want to hold your prem in continuous skin-to-skin contact, it will also work to ask a relative or close friend to take turns in holding her in skin-to-skin contact.

> **Important**: If you need to leave the ward, your prem can be left warmly wrapped in a bed <u>only</u> if she is able to maintain a stable body temperature on her own. Below 1800g, an infant needs to be warmed as she cannot do this for herself.

The staff can give you advice, and are there to support you and teach you according to the specific needs of your baby. The nurses will help you to transfer her to your chest, especially if she needs respirators, monitors, etc. These cables and tubes can be taped together to make it easier to work with them.

When to do skin-to-skin contact (SSC)

Skin-to-skin contact should be given to every baby at birth.

It is even more important for premature babies to help them stabilise (4).

Many places will only allow SSC once your prem is "stable", a particular weight and off all monitors and machines. This is a problem as babies quickly stabilise in skin-to-skin contact but they can take days to stabilise in an incubator.

You can do skin-to-skin contact when you are sleeping, or walking around.

You can do skin-to-skin contact with a baby on a ventilator or other machines (5).

Some countries use skin-to-skin contact or Kangaroo Care only as an add-on to incubator care as a bit of cuddling for 10-60 minutes a day. This helps mum and baby to bond together and does help the mother produce more breast milk (6)! Unfortunately, if you hold your baby for less than an hour or less than one full sleep awake cycle, it is of no benefit to her (7).

Skin-to-skin contact should ideally be 24 hours a day so that your baby is never separated from you, her Mum (8). (The ideal is for mum and dad to take it in turns for the full 24 hours!) In this way, her stress levels are kept as low as possible. Some hospitals do not have enough space for parents to sleep in the hospital, but now that you know how important it is that her brain wires properly, you will make it a priority to spend as much time as possible with her (9).

Take leave, get home help or do whatever is needed to give your prem your support – she is fighting for her life and she needs you to help her. You will never regret this time that you spend with her.

Can you still do skin-to-skin contact when your baby is jaundiced?

Hospitals have routinely left babies in incubators under ultraviolet light to correct their bilirubin levels if they look "yellow." This is needed for the baby but is often a lonely and worrying time for the parents who are told that they cannot hold their baby. There are ways to change this. Some places have bilirubin blankets so that the baby can be on mother and get the ultraviolet from a pad on her back. Other places can put dark covers over baby's eyes, and give baby ultraviolet treatment on mum's chest, with both under the lights. If we understand the importance of not separating Mum and baby there can always be creative solutions.

Babies getting phototherapy on mum.

> The smaller the prem, the more she needs her mother's chest to stabilise even if she needs medical technology as well. (See fine print page reference 4)

Details of the benefits of skin-to-skin contact

There are many benefits for the baby.

Babies stabilize faster when cared for in skin-to-skin contact than in incubators (See Ref (4)). (Babies do not stabilize as well in the incubator in the first six hours of

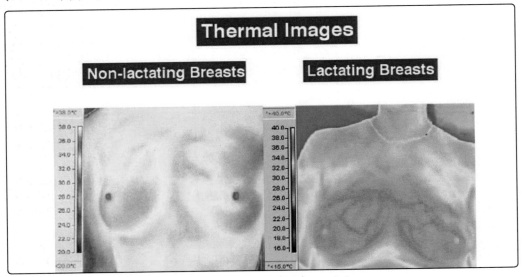

Ref: Peter Hartman used with permission.

life). Contact with a parent's skin helps the baby to maintain a more even temperature, heart rate, oxygen saturation and metabolism (10). The temperature on the chest of a breastfeeding mother is 2°C higher than that of a non-lactating mother (11). The mother's core temperature will automatically rise to warm a cold infant and drop to cool a hot infant. Studies have shown that the two breast temperatures can act independently in the case of twins of different temperatures! (12) Adjustment to life outside the womb is one of the most challenging times of change, and this is made safer by skin-to-skin contact. The benefits are faster weight gain and better and deeper sleep without the baby going into the deep apnoea sleep – this is when the main growth occurs (3). Fewer stress hormones are released in connection with the handling necessary for care. These stress hormones contribute to brain bleeds in premature infants.

The babies are stimulated to breastfeed as they can smell the mothers' milk. The skin-to-skin contact between mother and baby stimulates oxytocin production which increases milk production (13).

Breast milk production is stimulated by skin-to-skin care. The baby gets all the benefits of breast milk, including the correct milk for humans. (Formula is made with cows' milk which is designed for baby calves. The main protein in cows' milk, casein, is actually toxic to the human baby's gut leading to milk allergies on formula.)

The babies can breastfeed more often in skin-to-skin contact (SSC) as it encourages demand feeding. This is necessary for growth as the prem baby's stomach is very small at birth. The baby smells the breast milk straight away so the rooting instinct clicks in quickly and there are fewer problems with breastfeeding later. When the baby latches on to the breast correctly, there is less breast engorgement and the mother's nipples are not as sore. If the baby is premature, she also gets gestation-specific breast milk on the mother's chest, The milk content varies according to the baby's needs. The breast milk contains all the nucleotides necessary for brain growth.

> **In terms of protection, there will be fewer infections as the mum in the NICU will produce antibodies to the natural bacteria in the NICU and pass these antibodies onto her baby through the breast milk (14). The baby will get antibodies and about a thousand other protective factors from her mother's milk. The mother's colostrum carries the antibodies needed to protect the newborn with immunity. There are fewer long-term health problems for babies that have breastfed and had skin-to-skin contact; there are also fewer allergies (15).**

Faster growth: In skin-to-skin contact, the baby is in a relaxed mode so all her hormones prepare her gut to absorb food maximally. SSC babies can grow at 30g per day which is twice the rate of an incubator baby (2). Skin-to-skin care will mean less time in hospital (16).

A major benefit of skin-to-skin care is that the babies cry less so they have less stress hormones circulating (e.g. somatostatin and high levels of cortisol) (17). Somatostatin shuts down the gut and slows growth. Cortisol increases blood pressure and contributes to brain bleeds which are very common in premature infants.

In skin-to-skin contact, the **development** of the baby is the best. The baby is in the right place and therefore has the right behaviour. Skin-to-skin contact helps the baby to self-regulate and organize her systems. Without the presence of mother, the baby cannot bring her stress hormones down or get her brain to produce oxytocin to relax herself. The physical contact of co-sleeping or skin-to skin-care helps the baby to regulate her brain's stress response system (18).

The small movements of her mother's chest and hearing her heartbeat remind the baby to breathe so there is less apnoea.

Bonding: The baby is emotionally secure in skin-to-skin contact and the mother-infant bond is established early. This will mean that the baby will have better long term emotional stability. The primary bond of mother and child is the base on which all later relationships are built. There is increased intimacy and attachment and eye contact between mum and baby (19). SSC is especially good for mothers who experience difficult births or postnatal depression, for fathers and adoptive parents.

The developmental pathways of the brain grow best without stress. Learning is helped because of periods of quiet awareness. Rapid eye movement (REM) and non-REM sleep are both needed for memory formation. (See the section on protecting sleep).

Skin-to-skin contact has many benefits for you as her mother.

> **When a baby is born too early, the mother often feels helpless. Holding your baby in skin-to-skin contact will empower you to be part of the caring team and feel that you are able to really help your baby.**
>
> **Feelings of trauma at her early birth or the feelings of guilt at not carrying your baby to full term are eased by skin-to-skin contact.**
>
> **When you are close to your tiny baby, you will feel calmer (both parents); skin-to-skin contact allows you to give closeness and security to your child. Positive feelings for your baby strengthen as you care for her, and closeness helps you to interpret your baby's small signals, for example when she is waking up and ready to breastfeed.**

Skin–to-skin care at birth helps you to bond with your baby immediately; it also releases oxytocin, making you calmer and helping to start the production of breast milk. Skin-to-skin care can increase your milk supply as holding your baby close can stimulate the production of milk. Breastfeeding releases hormones which help to contract your womb, resulting in less blood loss right after delivery. The skin-to-skin contact helps you and your baby to settle into a rhythm of sleeping and waking together – "sleep synchrony" – so you both actually get more sleep.

Mothers often have a sense of guilt and anxiety when they deliver their babies prematurely and are prone to post-natal depression. Holding your baby on your chest in skin-to-skin contact helps you to feel that she is completing her gestation and that you are giving her the best possible care.

Carrying your prem baby in skin-to-skin contact means that you are able to be mobile sooner and can leave the hospital earlier. You will also be able to return to normal daily life sooner. (Having your baby tied firmly and safely on your chest in skin-to-skin contact will make a huge difference when you get home as you can do chores while still giving your baby the best care.)

Observing the benefits

	Date first seen
For your baby	
Her heart rate stabilizes on SSC.	
Her oxygen saturation improves on SSC.	
Her temperature is more stable.	
She cries less in SSC.	
She seems more peaceful.	
She sleeps better in SSC.	
She has less apnoea attacks in SSC.	
She has been able to start breastfeeding.	
She grows faster on the days she has more SSC.	
For mum	
You feel more peaceful and calm in SSC.	
You feel a closer bond to your baby.	
You can sleep when your baby sleeps.	
You get more sleep.	
You can read her tiny stress cues more easily.	
You can breastfeed more easily.	
You feel empowered and competent to care for your baby.	
You feel less fearful or guilty.	
You seem to have more breast milk.	
You feel more normal, and less like a patient.	
You feel that you can cope better.	
You feel more hopeful for the future.	

Fine Print Page – Skin-to-Skin Contact

This chapter addresses SSC for the parent: the references here support the statements and claims made. It is a long chapter, and so there are two fine print pages !!!!

1. Righard describes the natural birth behaviour, available as a video from www.geddesproduction.com . This research is also described by Widstrom (1987)
2. The KangaCarrier technique described in this chapter was developed and tested in a situation without incubators, by both authors and midwife Agneta Jurisoo, and provides safe 24 hour care. It was also tested in a RCT, see below. It frees mother's arms so as to allow safe sleep and also being able to stand and walk, within limits of IV lines and monitoring equipment.
3. The importance of sleep cycling is one of the key findings of recent neuroscience, and this paper describes the effect on SSC on sleep cycling. The advice given here is based on this.
4. The RCT by Bergman, Linley and Fawcus looked directly at comparing stabilisation. ALL babies 1200g to 2200g stabilised by 6 hours in SSC, only half those in incubators, the smaller the babies were, the more unstable they were in the incubator. Approximately 200 trials comparing SSC and incubator have all shown SSC to be as good or better … but because incubator is still assumed to be normal, SSC is now merely accepted. Actually, both from biology and neuroscience, SSC is normal, and the separation of the incubator makes the baby worse, it dysregulates the normal physiology.
5. Having said that SSC is better than incubator, very small babies still need the technology that supports immature respiratory function! None of the technology currently used in intensive care units is a contraindication to doing SSC. Obviously, SSC must be practised safely and with experience, and with due protocol. This paper describes some specific issues in doing so. Where experience is lacking and equipment unsuitable, SSC may not be advisable. A number of medical complications (e.g. gastroschisis, meningomyelocele) may also make SSC ill-advised.
6. In this rather old study, mothers did only 10 minutes of SSC a day, and yet it almost doubled their milk production. SSC allows increased suckling opportunity with hormones improving milk production, and enhances relaxation and parasympathetic stimulation.
7. Short periods may be good for mum, but not for baby. This study giving 20 min of SSC for extreme low birth weight babies "showed neither benefit or harm", and the authors do not recommend the "extra trouble and resources required". 20 minutes is too little !! Less than one sleep cycle does not allow for a sleep cycle, and is not recommended! There are a few other studies with similar results.
8. The "Kangaroo Mother Care" as defined by the World Health Organisation (WHO) advises continuous SSC, starting as early as possible, and also includes exclusive breastfeeding.
9. The WHO guide also provides practical guidelines for implementing and practising SSC.
10. This article summarise much of the broader aspects of the physiological benefits.
11. The higher skin temperature means this is the biological extra-uterine habitat for newborns
12. Mother's chest controls infant temperature in a narrow and stable range.
13. Uvnas-Moberg provides a review of the hormonal effects, includes pacifier effects.
14. In this careful prospective study, being fed infant formula increased infections from 29% (mother's milk fed) to 47%, and serious infections increased likewise: 19.5% vs 32.6%.
15. This recent WHO report provides the latest evidence on benefits, it is now firmly established that breastfeeding and mother's milk are superior, and formula is harmful.
16. In this study, premature babies got just 2 hours SSC starting when they were 1500g, they grew 3g a day faster, and they went home two days earlier.
17. This second article discussing somatostatin makes more direct links to SSC.
18. These comments are based on an interpretation of Schore's work, and other researchers (Teicher, Perry), and extrapolated in ongoing research to newborns.
19. Klaus and Kennell's work on "bonding" was discredited at the time, but is in fact supported by the most recent neuroscience.
20. Finally, here is the first review on KC, which is still valid, by Anderson (20).
21. The latest Cochrane review, updated 2008 (21).

There about 200 studies looking at specific outcomes, (temperature, heart rate, oxygen saturation etc), and Susan Ludington in Cleveland keeps an up to date inventory of these, older versions are available on www. kangaroomothercare.com

Reference List

(1)   Righard L, Alade MO. Effect of delivery room routines on success of first breast-feed. Lancet 1990 November 3;336(8723):1105-7.
(2)   Bergman NJ, Jurisoo LA. The 'kangaroo-method' for treating low birth weight babies in a developing country. Trop Doct 1994 April;24(2):57-60.

(3) Ludington-Hoe Sm, Johnson MW, Morgan K, Lewis T, Gutman J, Wilson D et al. Neurophysiologic assessment of neonatal sleep organization: Preliminary results of a randomized, controlled trial of skin contant with preterm infants. Pediatrics 2006 May;112(5):e909-e923.

(4) Bergman NJ, Linley LL, Fawcus SR. Randomized controlled trial of skin-to-skin contact from birth versus conventional incubator for physiological stabilization in 1200- to 2199-gram newborns. Acta Paediatr 2004 June;93(6):779-85.

(5) Ludington-Hoe Sm, FC, SJ, .Ceccardi JJ. Safe Criteria and Procedure for Kangaroo Care with Intubated Preterm Infants. JOGNN: Journal of Obstetric, Gynecologic, & Neonatal Nursing 2003 September;32(5):579-88.

(6) Hurst NM, Valentine CJ, Renfro L, Burns P, Ferlic L. Skin-to-skin holding in the neonatal intensive care unit influences maternal milk volume. J Perinatol 1997 May;17(3):213-7.

(7) Miles R, Cowan F, Glover V, Stevenson J, Modi N. A controlled trial of skin-to-skin contact in extremely preterm infants. Early Human Development 2006 July;82(7):447-55.

(8) Cattaneo A, Davanzo R, Bergman N, Charpak N. Kangaroo mother care in low-income countries. International Network in Kangaroo Mother Care. J Trop Pediatr 1998 October;44(5):279-82.

(9) WHO. Kangaroo mother care - a practical guide. WHO; 2003.

(10) Ludington-Hoe SM, Swinth JY. Developmental aspects of kangaroo care. J Obstet Gynecol Neonatal Nurs 1996 October;25(8):691-703.

(11) Bauer K, Pasel K, Versmold H. Chest skin temperature of mothers of term and preterm infants is higher than that of men and women. Pediatric Research 39[4], part2-195A. 1996.
Ref Type: Journal (Full)

(12) Ludington-Hoe Sm, Lewis T, Morgan K, Cong X, Anderson L, Reese S. Breast-infant temperature synchrony with twins during shared kangaroo care. JOGNN 2006;35(2):1-9.

(13) Uvnas-Moberg K, Eriksson M. Breastfeeding: physiological, endocrine and behavioural adaptations caused by oxytocin and local neurogenic activity in the nipple and mammary gland. Acta Paediatr 1996 May;85(5):525-30.

(14) Hylander MA, Strobino DM, Dhanireddy R. Human milk feedings and infection among very low birth weight infants. Pediatrics 1998 September;102(3):E38.

(15) WHO. Systematic reviews: Evidence on the long-term effects of breastfeeding. WHO 2007.

(16) Hann M, Malan A, Kronson M, Bergman N, Huskisson J. Kangaroo mother care. S Afr Med J 1999 January;89(1):37-9.

(17) Uvnas-Moberg K, Widstrom AM, Marchini G, Winberg J. Release of GI hormones in mother and infant by sensory stimulation. Acta Paediatr Scand 1987 November;76(6):851-60.

(18) Schore AN. Dysregulation of the right brain: a fundamental mechanism of traumatic attachment and the psychopathogenesis of posttraumatic stress disorder. Aust N Z J Psychiatry 2002 February;36(1):9-30.

(19) Klaus MH, Kennell JH. Maternal infant bonding. St Louis MO: CV Mosby; 1976.

(20) Anderson GC. An overview of research data and descriptive reports in the English language on kangaroo care, 1983- 1991. Journal of Perinatology X1[3], 218-226. 1991.
Ref Type: Magazine Article

(21) Moore ER, Anderson GC, Bergman N. Early skin-to-skin contact for mothers and their healthy newborn infants. Cochrane Database of Systematic Reviews 2008;(4).

56

BREAST MILK AND BREASTFEEDING

> Mum, do ALL you possibly can to express milk for
> your prem baby.
> No one else can do this for her.

1   Breast milk

▶ is the right food for your baby's brain to grow.

▶ Your prem baby needs breast milk even more than a full term baby.

▶ Your baby needs colostrum to protect her gut.

▶ has FAR more benefits than formula.

▶ is dynamic; it is produced for your specific baby at her specific stage of development.

2   Ways of feeding prem babies

▶ By TPN (Total Parenteral nutrition, ie intravenous feeding)

▶ By NGT or OGT (naso- or oro-gastric tube

▶ By cup

▶ By breastfeeding

3   Breastfeeding your prem

▶ "Breast feeding is normal".

▶ Breastfeeding provides the right sensations for brain-wiring.

▶ If you want to breastfeed, start expressing straight away.

▶ When you hold your baby in skin-to-skin contact, you will produce more breast milk.

▶ The more often your baby feeds, the more breast milk is produced.

▶ From 28 weeks gestation onwards, a prem is able to suckle on the breast.

> Breast fed is normal, accept no substitutes.

The stomach of a prem is tiny, so she will prefer to be fed small amounts often (every 60-90minutes).

Bottle feeding is stressful for a baby.

1 BREASTMILK

> **Firstly: your baby's brain needs the correct food: breast milk.**

This section is valid for ALL babies. Later we will focus specifically on premature babies.

Look at this amazing list of benefits of breast milk and you will see why it is so important to give your baby your breast milk (1). It is one of the most important things that you as a mother can do for your baby, to give her health now and in the future.

MORE BENEFITS of Breast milk

▶ Baby gets the best food for growth, especially for brain growth.

▶ Baby gets antibodies to protect against and to fight infections.

▶ Better health

▶ Breast milk changes to meet the baby's specific needs

▶ Better bone density

FEWER PROBLEMS

▶ less sickness and time in hospital;

▶ less diahorrea and vomiting;

▶ less gastroenteritis;

▶ less necrotizing enterocolitis (NEC, a nasty kind of gut infection);

▶ less colic;

▶ less childhood diabetes or obesity;

▶ fewer ear infections;

▶ fewer respiratory infections (pneumonia, bronchitis etc);

▶ fewer allergies, less asthma;

▶ less septicaemia (blood poisoning);

▶ less Sudden Infant Death Syndrome (SIDS, cot death);

▶ less meningitis;

▶ less appendicitis;

▶ less tooth decay;

▶ reduced risk of heart disease later in life;

▶ reduced risk of Vitamin E and iron deficiencies.

What milk? Breast milk!

Humans are mammals. That word means that they breastfeed their babies with their own milk. The "Professional Advice" that tells mothers not to exclusively breastfeed is not based on science! There is now overwhelming evidence that mother's own milk (MOM) is the best food for babies (see fine print page) (1;2). Sometimes it takes a while before hospitals change what they do with new evidence. Often doctors and hospitals say formula is the only option for prems, because it is easier or more convenient for them.

Mum: make every effort to produce milk and make sure your baby gets the best, your milk!

▶ **The very best food for your baby is your milk.**

▶ **Mother's milk is the right food for the baby's brain.**

▶ **Breastfeeding provides the right sensations for brain-wiring.**

Breast milk changes throughout the tiny baby's life and is different from birth to a week, to a month, to a year. **Breast milk is dynamic; it is produced for that specific baby at that specific stage of development.** It will be thinner if it is hot and the baby many need extra fluids. It changes through the day (3).

You may have heard the slogan, "Breast is best". This implies that formula is OK.

"Breast feeding is normal" is more accurate.

Putting it this way tells you that anything else is abnormal, and therefore worse! Your baby needs normal good food, not abnormal replacement. Breast milk is the only right milk for the human baby. It has over a thousand different components which the baby needs (4). Formula has only 30! All formula companies know that breast milk is the "gold standard", and try to copy it. That should tell you just how valuable breast milk is! Formula can never be as good as breast milk. Artificial formula comes from cows that produce milk designed for calves that eat grass and have 4 stomachs. Formula is abnormal for human babies! It has even been suggested that formula should only be allowed on prescription!

Cow's milk is not right for human babies!! (5)…. This diagram shows that cows' milk is 90% casein, (8% in human milk). Casein is a foreign protein which is toxic to the human baby's stomach. Cow casein is very different from human casein (it may be that this contributes to colic). This is even more of a problem if the baby is premature.

Human milk is 25% NPN, (non-protein nitrogen) (3); these are 200 or more different tiny proteins ready for building the human baby's brain and gut, and providing immune protection. Cow's milk has only 2% of these NPNs! Two thirds of human milk protein is "whey", which contains immune protection factors, like antibodies.

So – is this information on breastmilk relevant for your PREMATURE baby?

Absolutely! (6)

Prem babies need breast milk even more than full term babies

Prems are often unable to keep their fluid balance right. Prems dry out very quickly through the very thin skin and through their lungs. Their bodies are 90% water, so one of the big challenges is to get enough fluid into your baby, and also to get enough food, not just for survival, but to actively grow.

Your tiny prem may desperately need the fluids and nutrition while your breast milk is starting so the NICU staff may give her other food. Total Parenteral Nutrition (TPN) is often given intravenously, as a temporary measure until you can give breast milk. (I will say a little more in the next chapter.)

It is very important to give the early breast milk called colostrum (7). Even two drops of this "watery" first milk given to the baby as soon as possible after birth are vital. Colostrum has surface antibodies that protect the stomach lining, plus a host of other protective factors. That is why it is called "white gold".

Every baby needs colostrum to protect the gut.
Even one "top up" feed of formula will disturb the gut of the newborn for life!

The baby's metabolism will adapt better if she is breastfed, than if she is artificially fed. It is also better if she is exclusively breastfed than if she has mixed feeds (some breast, some formula) (8).

Formula fed prems have a 6–9 times increase in necrotising enterocolitis (NEC).

Any of your breast milk that you can supply to your baby is important, specifically for her brain growth. (See the chapter on neuroscience.)
Babies need only breast milk for brain growth.

Breast milk contains long- and medium-chain fatty acids (called omega 6 and 3). These fats make myelin, which coats the nerves and acts like insulation around an electric cord. This makes messages in the brain go faster, an important part of future intelligence (9). It is correct to say that breast milk increases intelligence! (10) Nothing else can do this for the brain. Interestingly, the fat content of the mother's milk increases over the first year, when the myelin is needed in the brain. (11)

The baby's brain is the most important organ being developed in the last ten weeks of pregnancy. If the baby is born too early, the mother's body automatically produces in her breast milk what her prem baby would have received via the umbilical cord and what she needs for her brain to grow properly,. Mother's milk is "gestation–specific". That is, the food in the breast milk of a 27 week gestation baby is different from the food for a baby of 31 weeks gestation, which is different from the food for a full term baby. The contents of the milk are different for each breastfeeding premature baby to supply the individual needs of that specific baby at that time.

Expressing breast milk

The next important thing is how to get this milk!

> ### Almost every mother is able to produce breast milk.

It is important to express milk because you are providing your baby with the best nutrition; nutrition that no-one else can duplicate at a critical time in her life. It may take extra time and hard work to express milk, but as you have read – it is well worth the effort. Breast milk is the best food for your baby's brain. You may want to invest in the help of a supportive lactation consultant to help get your milk production going – it is really worthwhile (6).

Hand expressing

If your baby has delivered normally, your body will have started producing hormones like prolactin to start the production of milk, and oxytocin to release it. Skin-to-skin contact aids the release of these hormones, which is another reason why it is so essential!!

Start expressing milk at birth or within 6 hours. Remember that those first few drops of colostrum are important to protect your baby's stomach. You can express your breast milk <u>by hand</u> or you can use <u>a pump</u> to get your milk going. If you are using a pump, put cream on the nipple so that it does not hurt. Start on the lowest setting for 5 minutes a side every 2–3 hours during the day and 3–4 hourly at night. It is better to pump often and for short times to get the milk started. By the second day you can pump for 10 minutes at a time. You may feel anxious that you have to produce enough milk, but your baby needs less in the first few days. It will be easier to pump milk if you can see or touch your baby while pumping. Your milk will increase in volume the more you pump and by two weeks you should aim for at least 500 ml per day, the more the better. This is more than your baby needs now, but you will need it for the future. You can store it or donate it to a milk bank (to help another mum who may be struggling.)

> ### If you do want to breastfeed, start expressing straight away.

If you **hold your baby in skin-to-skin contact, more milk will be produced,** your baby will be calmer, and should latch better. Carry her skin-to-skin for 15 to 30 minutes before a feed. This will calm you and your baby! Hormones are released in your baby to prepare her gut to receive the milk, and in you that assist in the let-down reflex.

Expressed Breast Milk (EBM) can be safely stored for

▶ 4 hours in a cool room;

▶ 24 hours in a fridge (<4°C);

▶ 2 weeks in a freezer compartment;

▶ 3 months in a freezer.

<u>Important</u>: This milk needs to be carefully labelled with your name and the date and time.

> **Plan before birth (if you read this then!) to give your baby colostrum.**
> **Express milk for your baby as soon after birth as you can.**
> **Express milk as frequently as possible.**
> **Keep expressing to get your milk flowing.**

For mums

How much milk could you produce first day? ....

Second day? ....

Third day ? ....

End of week 1 ....

Now that we know that it is essential to give your prem breast milk, let us look at how to get it into her!

Fine Print Page – Breastmilk and Breastfeeding

There are more breastfeeding references in the next two chapters!

1   Policy statement from American Academy of Paediatrics updated recommendations on breastfeeding, summarises evidence at 2005, which has increased since then.
2.   World Health Organisation systematic review on long term effects, shows breastfeeding improves blood pressure, cholesterol, overweight, schooling and IQ.
3.   Milk volume is shown to be directly determined by infant demand, other factors also, see also ref 5.
4.   There are a whole variety of different immune systems and mechanisms, and they act synergistically. One single group alone, the glycans, has several thousand different varieties.
5.   This article highlights differences between human and cows milk in all aspects. (For more on NPN see Rudloff & Kunz 1997).
6.   This article summarises benefits specific to premature infants, and then gives general advice on how to ensure feeding by mothers' own milk can be adopted by neonatal units.
7.   Reviews development of the gut in relation to colostrum, there are other functions of colostrum also! Dr Sears writes that one drop of milk contains one million active immunity cells.
8.   Exclusive really means nothing else … complementary feeding is harmful.
9.   One single gene, FADS2, will make for a 6 – 8 point increase in IQ if it can have the triglyceride in mother's milk and make it into myelin.
10. The debate about breastfeeding and intelligence is over. BUT there are other important things to do over and above breastfeeding to enhance development.
11. Up to 6 months, milk is 7.4% fat, but at 12 months it is 10.7% (nearly 50% more). It might not be major for calorie requirement, but it is not used as fuel calories, it is used in the brain.

Reference List

(1)   Gartner LM, Morton J, Lawrence RA, Naylor AJ, O'Hare D, Schanler RJ et al. Breastfeeding and the use of human milk. Pediatrics 2005 February;115(2):496-506.
(2)   WHO. Systematic reviews: Evidence on the long-term effects of breastfeeding. WHO 2007.
(3)   Picciano MF. Human milk: nutritional aspects of a dynamic food. Biol Neonate 1998;74(2):84-93.
(4)   Xanthou M. Immune protection of human milk. Biol Neonate 1998;74(2):121-33.
(5)   Emmett PM, Rogers IS. Properties of human milk and their relationship with maternal nutrition. Early Hum Dev 1997 October 29;49 Suppl:S7-S28.
(6)   Schanler RJ. Suitability of human milk for the low-birthweight infant. Clinics in Perinatology 1995 March;22(1):207-22.
(7)   Xu RJ. Development of the newborn GI tract and its relation to colostrum/milk intake: a review. Reprod Fertil Dev 1996;8(1):35-48.
(8)   Habicht JP. Expert consultation on the optimal duration of exclusive breastfeeding: the process, recommendations, and challenges for the future. Adv Exp Med Biol 2004;554:79-87.:79-87.
(9)   Caspi A, Williams B, Kim-Cohen J, Craig IW, Milne BJ, Pouldon R et al. Moderation of breastfeeding effects on the IQ by genetic variation in fatty acid metabolism. PNAS 2007;104(47):18860-5.
(10) Kramer MS, Aboud F, Mironova E, Vanilovich I, Platt RW, Matush L et al. Breastfeeding and child cognitive development: new evidence from a large randomized trial. Archives Of General Psychiatry 2008 May;65(5):578-84.
(11) Mandel D, Lubetzky R, Dollberg S, Barak S, Mimouni FB. Fat and Energy Contents of Expressed Human Breast Milk in Prolonged Lactation. Pediatrics 2005 September 1;116(3):e432-e435.

WAYS OF FEEDING PREM BABIES

Prem babies need breast milk even more than full term babies!

Feeding you prem will depend on your own baby's needs, development and situation. It will also depend on your hospital's methods and policies.

Do insist on breast milk as far as you possibly can!

Also, avoid bottle feeding if you possibly can – see why further down!!.

For an extremely premature baby, there is a usual progression, and I shall explain these steps:

TPN ⟶ NGT/OGT ⟶ finger feed ⟶ cup feed ⟶ breastfeed

"TPN" stands for Total Parenteral Nutrition, and means feeding your baby directly into the blood, through an intravenous line, bypassing the stomach. This is done when the gut is just too immature (usually less than 28 weeks) to be able to digest your milk. Though this is difficult and expensive, it is often necessary and life saving. But, as I said earlier, do start expressing your milk in the meantime! The colostrum is still safe to give.

My baby did not need   TPN _____

My baby did need TPN: started _____ (date)

                         Ended _____

                         Reason _____

How to feed your prem breast milk

In the previous chapter we looked at how to express milk. At 28 weeks of gestation your baby may struggle to latch onto the breast and may need your breast milk through a tube into the stomach.

- A **nasogastric tube (NGT)** goes through the nose directly into the gut, and

- an **orogastric tube (OGT)** goes through the mouth straight to the stomach.

- There are reasons for both.

To get breastfeeding going, express two drops of milk for your prem to smell. Let her suckle on the breast at the same time as you have the tube in her nose or mouth.

OGT/NGT feeding

Cup-feeding: you may need to cup-feed, or feed your milk in a teaspoon (1). Avoid using a bottle as it is stressful for your baby. The nurses can <u>cup feed</u> or spoon feed your milk when you are not there.

If the baby is struggling to suck, a syringe can be put into the side of her mouth while on the breast.

To encourage sucking, you can try **"finger-feeding"** where a very fine tube is taped onto your finger, to teach her sucking skills.

What about bottle feeding?

Cup feeding

Many hospitals use bottles to feed the babies as it is convenient for the nurses, and they can know exactly how much food the baby has had. But bottle-feeding is stressful for any baby as she cannot co-ordinate the muscles she uses for sucking and breathing (2). Some of the muscles for sucking from a bottle are the same muscles used for breathing. (Try blocking your nose, swallowing from a straw and breathing at the same time!) So your baby sucks from the bottle until she runs out of air, then she breathes and rests, then she sucks some more.

A baby also gets too much milk, too fast from a bottle. This is not helpful to her (3).

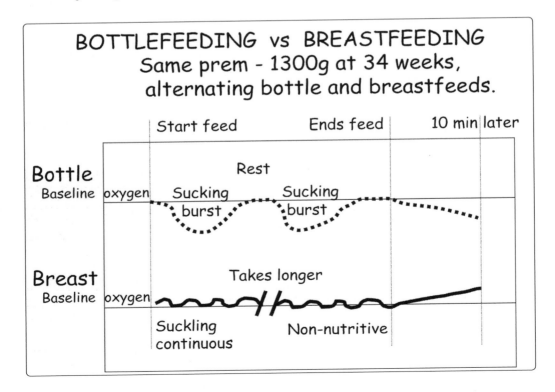

<u>Important</u> - suck and suckle are not the same.
Suckling is more like a chewing motion using the jaw.
Babies can suckle from a breast and breathe at the same time!

Some nurses may believe that suckling from a breast is more tiring for the baby, and so recommend the bottle. Actually, bottle feeding is more stressful and breastfeeding uses less energy (4).

What about pacifiers or "dummies"?

Pacifiers are often used to calm a crying baby, which is helpful if you cannot be there. It is important that tiny babies do not cry so that their stress levels are not increased. Pacifiers are often used as a compromise (5;6). If mother and baby are kept together, babies should not need to cry!

Pacifiers also stimulate the vagus nerve, which helps the stomach empty faster. This is not helpful as the baby's tummy should not empty too quickly (7).

Pacifiers are discouraged in international "Baby Friendly Hospitals", for good reasons. Like the nipple or teat of a bottle, the nipple of a pacifier is often too hard and too big for a premature baby. Bottles and pacifiers use a sucking method which uses cheek muscles instead of the jaw muscles used in breastfeeding. Sucking on a pacifier or bottle strengthens the wrong muscles and the baby cannot latch onto the nipple properly. The result may be that the mother gets cracked, sore nipples.

The cheek development is also not good for later speech development. As humans, we speak with our jaw muscles, not our cheek muscles.

Pacifiers can also cause dental deformation, as the teeth can be pushed crookedly in the jaw. When a baby is sucking on a pacifier or bottle while lying flat, saliva collects in the back of the mouth. This fluid may run into the Eustachian tube, which can cause middle ear infections.

I know that the use of pacifiers is a sensitive issue, but as parents you should be given the information and be allowed to make your own choices.

How much and how often to feed a fullterm baby?

How babies are fed varies enormously from hospital to hospital. Let us first look at a full term baby, then at how your prem should feed.

The "daily amount required" for a baby to grow is known, and is about 160 ml of milk per kilogram of weight per day. The average **full-term newborn** weighs about 3 kg, so let us use 480 ml (3 kg x 160 ml) as the daily amount required. When the baby comes home and is feeding three hourly, she needs 60 ml each time. The problem is that there is no research evidence to show that this is the size of the stomach. The research available suggests that the stomach size is only about 20 ml – that is only 2 tablespoons! (8–10) It means that the baby really needs to feed once every hour and take a smaller amount.

The stomach is elastic, and can stretch. It behaves a bit like a balloon; when you stretch it several times, it loses its ability to shrink back to the normal small size, and becomes bigger. Are we stretching our babies' stomachs too much? (Imagine your own discomfort after eating too big a meal.)

When the baby breastfeeds, she stimulates the breast with rapid mouth movements to produce a "milk ejection reflex". The volume of this is 30 mls at most, in all mothers, no matter how big or small their breasts are. Research has also shown that babies do not swallow the whole reflex and the breast stores the remaining amount for later (11;12).

The "one hourly feeding schedule" also matches other biological behaviours. The stomach empties a milk meal in 60 minutes. Also, the normal sleep cycle of a baby is approximately 60 minutes. The sugar content of milk lasts just 60 minutes. The proteins in milk come in very low concentration, so they also need topping up every hour.

As a mother, I can hear you say that feeding once every hour would be far too demanding. Actually, and surprisingly, it is much easier, quicker and saves time!

A "normal" breastfeeding session (meaning one dose every three hours) takes about 20 to 25 minutes. This is because the baby has to stimulate four or five ejection reflexes in succession to get the milk she knows she needs. Let us leave aside the burping time and the comfort time, and just say it takes 20 minutes each time. If you do that 8 times a day, you spend about 3 hours feeding your baby.

Now, the very first ejection reflex takes less than 2 minutes for the baby to produce (11;13), and the baby can swallow it in about half a minute, without problems. Quick and easy: two and a half minutes, 24 times a day, is just one hour you have spent feeding your baby. You have saved yourself two hours, and you do not need to burp her, because the stomach is relaxed and able to deal with the air by itself.

How much and how often to feed your prem baby?

How does this apply to **premature** babies? Most hospitals start feeding extremely small babies once an hour, then every two hours and aim to send babies home feeding three hourly.

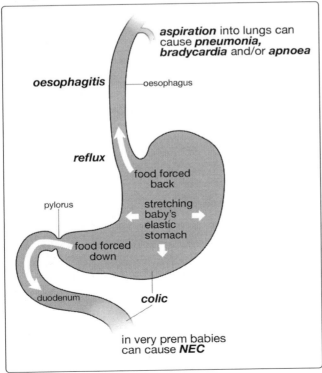

Problems caused by feeding baby too much.

Prems have very small stomachs, and the stomach size is proportional to the physical size of the baby. "Reflux" is common in premature babies; this happens when stomach contents go back up the oesophagus and cause burning pain(14). Apnoea may also be caused this way. In many hospitals, babies are routinely treated for this, even operated on. Everyone knows babies burp, or 'spit up" after a meal, and this has long been regarded as "normal". But is it necessary?

At the same time as excess milk comes back up as reflux, it goes right through the stomach into the small bowel, where it may also cause problems. This large volume may also be a cause of the colic that so many normal babies get.

> **A prem baby's stomach and body are more sensitive than those of a full term baby.**

The prem is less resilient and copes less well with stress. Babies who are fed small amounts frequently have less colic.

As the stomach empties in 60 minutes, the blood sugar level also starts to fall. Hospitals often do routine heel prick tests on newborn and premature babies to check for low blood sugar. The heel prick is a stressful and painful event for the baby, and calories are used for crying. This may be one reason why small babies grow so slowly. When the blood sugar level is low, the baby is given sugar water or extra sugar in the drip. You are told your baby is "hypoglycemic", but it could be better translated as "hungry"! (She had 24 hour continuous feeding inside you!) If your baby feeds frequently and has small amounts, she does not need this extra sugar.

> **There are good reasons to feed your prem baby once an hour.**

Nurses are often busy; your baby needs you, her mum, to be there to feed her <u>regularly</u>. Many prems do not grow well because they are not fed small amounts often enough. Prems in skin-to-skin contact often grow at the rate of 30g a day compared to 10g / day for a baby in an incubator. Feeding and holding your baby in skin-to-skin contact will shorten your stay in hospital because your baby will grow faster.

FOR MUMS:

My baby had a feeding tube   started .... (date)

                                  Ended ....

The tube was in the .... (nose, mouth)

I first finger fed my baby .... (date) at .... days old.

I first cup-fed my baby............................... (date) at .... days old.

I first BREASTFED my baby............................. (date) at .... days old. ☺

My NICU policy was to aim at.. (2 hourly, 3hourly, 4 hourly)

My baby got feeds at .... intervals

(Describe baby's comfort level after feeds)

....

....

....

....

....

....

....

....

....

....

....

....

....

....

....

....

Fine Print Page – Feeding Your Prem

1. This is a technical review, and covers cup-feeding evidence pages 4, and 62-64. It can be downloaded from internet: http://www.who.int/child_adolescent_health/documents/9241595094/en/index.html   and covers all aspects of feeding a low birth weight infant.

2. Babies were 32 weeks, and the same babies were studied bottle-feeding and breastfeeding. Bottle-feeding caused hypoxia.

3. Different muscles are used to suck from a bottle and suckle from a breast, despite a teat modified to resemble the breast nipple.

4. Quote "There were 2 episodes of apnea (breath pause more than 20 seconds) and 20 episodes of oxygen desaturation ($PaO_2 < 90\%$) during bottle-feeding and none during breastfeeding. We conclude that breastfeeding is a more physiological feeding method for the preterm infant and bottle-feeding may be more stressful."

5–7. There are benefits of pacifiers, but these have only been studied in the short term, not the long term. The effect on breastfeeding is however widely accepted, though hard to prove.

8. This paper describes the stomach growing as seen on ultrasound. It grows in proportion to the baby, and though a volume is not provided, the data can be used to calculate a volume of 12 mls before birth.

9. Very similar study, but shows full term fetus swallowing over 30 minutes to fill stomach to about 12 mls, and then gastric peristalsis emptying the stomach in about 5 – 10 minutes.

10. In this study, stillborn babies and those dying in the first week were studied, and the stomach stretched to full capacity with water pressure … volumes of about 15 – 20 mls. So unstretched it would be 12 ml !!!

11–12. This paper describes an ultrasound of a breast during feeding. The milk ejection reflex (MER) fills the ducts, and milk can be seen flowing out, but also back if not drunk by baby. The volume of the breast was measured, and varied greatly, depending on how much of the reflex the baby swallowed at that feed. The weight gain of the baby shows also the volume of milk produced, and is 30 mls for the first MER, and then 20ml or so for each subsequent, the whole feed taking 15 minutes.

13. here are many papers studying this, but this one shows nicely how very common reflux is. But it also shows the effects of feeding two hourly or three hourly or four hourly. Milk buffers acid, and so to get acid reflux, this only happens three hours after a milk meal. Babies that breastfed frequently may get reflux, but it is not acid reflux!!

Reference List

(1) Edmond KT, Bahl R. Optimal feeding of low-birth-weight infants technical review. WHO 2006;1-131.

(2) Meier P. Bottle- and breast-feeding: effects on transcutaneous oxygen pressure and temperature in preterm infants. Nursing Research 1988 January;37(1):36-41.

(3) Mizuno K, Fujimaki K, Sawada M. Sucking behavior at breast during the early newborn period affects later breast-feeding rate and duration of breast-feeding. Pediatrics International: Official Journal Of The Japan Pediatric Society 2004 February;46(1):15-20.

(4) Chen CH, Wang TM, Chang HM, Chi CS. The effect of breast - and bottle-feeding on oxygen saturation and body temperature in preterm infants. J Hum Lact 2000 February;16(1):21-7.

(5) Anderson GC. [Skin-to-skin: the kangaroo technic in western Europe]. Servir 1989 November;37(6):316-20.

(6) Pinelli J, Symington A. How rewarding can a pacifier be? A systematic review of nonnutritive sucking in preterm infants. Neonatal Netw 2000 December;19(8):41-8.

(7) Widstrom AM, Marchini G, Matthiesen AS, Werner S, Winberg J, Uvnas-Moberg K. Nonnutritive sucking in tube-fed preterm infants: effects on gastric motility and gastric contents of somatostatin. J Pediatr Gastroenterol Nutr 1988 July;7(4):517-23.

(8) Goldstein I, Reece EA, Yarkoni S, Wan M, Green JL, Hobbins JC. Growth of the fetal stomach in normal pregnancies. Obstet Gynecol 1987 October;70(4):641-4.

(9) Naveed M, Manjunath CS, Sreenivas, V. An autopsy Study of Relationship between Perinatal Stomach Capacity and Birth Weight. Indian J Gastroenterol 1992;11(4):156-8.

(10) Sase M, Miwa I, Sumie M, Nakata M, Sugino N, Okada K et al. Gastric emptying cycles in the human fetus. American Journal Of Obstetrics And Gynecology 2005 September;193(3 Pt 2):1000-4.

(11) Prime DK, Geddes DT, Hartmann PE. Oxytocin: Milk ejection and maternal-infant well-being. Hale & Hartmann's Textbook of Human Lactation 2007;141-55.

(12) Ramsay DT, Kent JC, Owens RA, Hartmann PE. Ultrasound Imaging of Milk Ejection in the Breast of Lactating Women. Pediatrics 2004 February;113(2):361-7.

(13) Lopez-Alonso M, Moya MJ, Cabo JA, Ribas J, M, Silny J et al. Twenty-four-hour esophageal impedance-pH monitoring in healthy preterm neonates: rate and characteristics of acid, weakly acidic, and weakly alkaline gastroesophageal reflux. Pediatrics 2006 August;118(2):e299-e308.

(14) Lopez-Alonso M, Moya MJ, Cabo JA, Ribas J, M, Silny J et al. Twenty-four-hour esophageal impedance-pH monitoring in healthy preterm neonates: rate and characteristics of acid, weakly acidic, and weakly alkaline gastroesophageal reflux. Pediatrics 2006 August;118(2):e299-e308.

BREASTFEEDING YOUR PREM

The huge benefits from exclusively breastfeeding from birth to 6 months are well-researched and proven (1;2). In the first section we looked at the benefits from the actual breast milk. The food is only a small part of what your baby is getting from you to help her grow.

The physical action of breastfeeding itself produces benefits and helps brain growth. All of the sensations that the baby receives in skin-to-skin contact together with the breast milk produce various types of intelligence.

Being in the right place on mum's chest and breastfeeding makes the brain grow best as the baby feels SAFE and LOVED (see the diagram "Sensations that Wire the Brain" in the first few hours chapter). By breastfeeding, you are wiring your baby's brain for health for her whole life and for intelligence.

Can tiny prems breastfeed?

Yes, they can!

This may seem surprising, but if we look at the capabilities of the premature baby, we see that prems are not as helpless as many believe.

From 28 weeks gestation onwards a prem baby <u>can</u> suckle on the breast (3-5).

If your baby is born prematurely, you need to have some idea of what she can do. Each baby is unique, so there will be variation according to how premature your baby was born.

Here is the basic biology of what your baby would be doing if she were still in your womb.

- ▶ By 18 – 24 weeks the baby inside her mum is able to swallow amniotic fluid.
- ▶ By 22 weeks she can pout her lips (so as to close her lips to get a seal when suckling).
- ▶ By full term a baby has practised all the breastfeeding behaviours for many weeks, and is ready to breastfeed.

When a baby is born prematurely, these behaviours are present but not well practised. The prem develops skills in the following order (5).

- ▶ By 28 weeks gestation she has a strong rooting reflex and is able to suck, swallow and breathe, but only briefly and these may not be co-ordinated.
- ▶ By 31 weeks, there is repeated swallowing of milk from the breast.
- ▶ By 30–32 weeks the baby is able to co-ordinate sucking, swallowing and breathing.
- ▶ By 34 weeks the baby can breastfeed fully.

Your baby has a strong gag reflex to protect her from getting milk down her airway (6). If she has been suctioned at birth or had a feeding tube, she may gag if anything, even the breast, is placed in her mouth (7;8). Go slowly and gently.

Keep your baby in the right <u>place</u> (in skin-to-skin contact) and she will show the right <u>behaviours</u>. These are called "rooting behaviours". As soon as she starts any of the following <u>pre-feeding cues</u> or signs, try putting her on the breast.

Pre-feeding cues

- ▶ licking her lips, mouth movements;
- ▶ turning her head towards your breast;
- ▶ smelling your nipple, touching it with her hands;
- ▶ nuzzling.

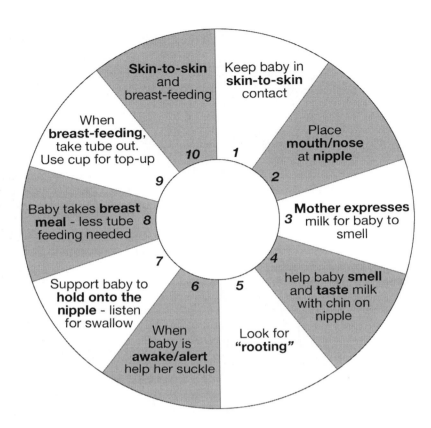

This wheel (adapted from Persson) describes the ten small steps to breast-feeding (9;10):

1   Baby must be in skin-to-skin contact.

2   Baby smells the nipple.

3   Baby smells the breast milk.

4   Baby tastes the breast milk on the nipple.

5   Baby will make mouth movements called rooting (prems may only sip the milk at first).

6   Baby must be awake and alert for suckling.

7   Baby latches on and swallows milk.

8   First breast milk meal. Steps 1–7 go fast for full term babies, prems may need successive alert times.

9   Baby feeds frequently, (for prems every 60–90 minutes).

10   Mum and baby are together continuously.

Mum, be encouraged if your baby is doing <u>any</u> of these tiny steps. Maybe you could write a date and time next to each one so that you can see her progress. Dad, you can be a wonderful help to your wife by encouraging her with breastfeeding. It may seem very slow and frustrating for her.

Here are some things that mum can do to encourage breastfeeding.

From outside the mouth, rub in small circles on the dimple area near your baby's mouth. Rub small circles also on the cheek where the baby's jaw bone connects to her skull.

Using your small finger, rub both these areas inside the mouth. Rub in small circles in the soft tissue just under her chin bone. This will stimulate the muscles used for breastfeeding. Encourage your baby to suck on her fist. Let her try to suckle on your nipple; even if she does not get it right, she is still collecting the right sensations to encourage breastfeeding behaviour.

Again, you may need to call in a lactation consultant or breastfeeding support person to help you to get your prem latching and breastfeeding properly. It may take time. There are MANY excellent books on breastfeeding so I will not go into more detail here (11).

As the baby suckles, the nipple is pulled deep into her mouth. The action of suckling stimulates the back of the mouth, the soft palate and soothes the baby as it aids the release of oxytocin. Because she is soothed and calmed, her gut will absorb all her food. You need to hold your baby "tummy to Mummy" and she needs a good amount of your areola or nipple inside her mouth for a proper latch. Try to relax and this will help your baby to relax as well. Listen for her swallowing to know that she is drinking properly.

> **The more often your baby feeds, the more milk is produced, so feed her small amounts often.**

Always put the baby next to your breast to taste and smell the nipple and milk even if it is only a drop. All newborns, even tiny prems, have a strong sense of smell. You want your baby to smell and taste the right and expected food and link it to you, her mum. Her small hands' kneading movements on your breasts, and her tiny attempts at suckling, will help towards your breasts producing her next meal.

Fine Print Page – Breastfeeding Your Premature

1. This statement is not generally believed … but the evidence has been building up over the years, and it is only recently that there is enough of it for the World Health Organisation to "put its head on the block" ! From abstract: "WHO (to) change … to a recommendation to promote exclusive breastfeeding for six months.". Further "The amount of scientific evidence available was more than is often available for policy decisions in health, but much less than desirable to address issues of generalizability across and within populations."

2. A Cochrane review allows only the strictest possible evidence criteria, and is therefore worded very cautiously. This paper chose only 20 best studies from 2688 articles, and ends by saying that bigger and better studies are needed to "confirm the health benefits reported thus far, and to investigate other potential effects on health and development, especially over the long term."

3–5. These papers introduce the work of Kerstin Hedberg-Nyqvist. Conclusion from Ref 5; "Very preterm infants have the capacity for early development of oral motor competence that it sufficient for establishment of full breastfeeding at a low postmenstrual age."

6. Authors define breastfeeding as the "physiological norm", during which "swallowing occurred nonrandomly between breaths and did not interfere with breathing."

7—8 . This is a review of routines, quote: "Many common care practices during labor, birth, and the immediate postpartum period impact the fetal to neonatal transition, including … suctioning protocols". And it summarises by "routine suctioning of infants at birth has not been found to be beneficial." Widstrom writes that the sequence of prefeeding behaviour described in the Skin-to-Skin Contact chapter "was disrupted in children who had undergone gastric suction."

9–10. Wahlberg first published "Persson's Wheel", more accessible version with the science explained is in Meier's chapter.

11. Biological Nurturing expands some of these concepts: http://www.biologicalnurturing.com/

Reference List

(1)   Habicht JP. Expert consultation on the optimal duration of exclusive breastfeeding: the process, recommendations, and challenges for the future. Adv Exp Med Biol 2004;554:79-87.:79-87.

(2)   Kramer MS, Kakuma R. The optimal duration of exclusive breastfeeding: a systematic review. Adv Exp Med Biol 2004;554:63-77.:63-77.

(3)   Nyqvist KH, Rubertsson C, Ewald U, Sjoden P. Development of the Preterm Infant Breastfeeding Behavior Scale (PIBBS): a study of nurse-mother agreement. J HUM LACT 1996 September;12(3):207-19.

(4)   Nyqvist KH, Sj+¦d+¬n PO, Ewald U. The development of preterm infants' breastfeeding behavior. Early Human Development 1999 July;55(3):247-64.

(5)   Nyqvist KH. Early attainment of breastfeeding competence in very preterm infants. Acta Paediatrica 2008 June;97(6):776-81.

(6)   Goldfield EC, Richardson MJ, Lee KG, Margetts S. Coordination of sucking, swallowing, and breathing and oxygen saturation during early infant breast-feeding and bottle-feeding. Pediatr Res 2006 October 28;60(4):450-5.

(7)   Mercer JS, Erickson-Owens DA, Graves B, Haley MM. Evidence-based practices for the fetal to newborn transition. Journal of Midwifery and Womens Health 2007;52(3):262-72.

(8)   Widstrom AM, Ransjo-Arvidson AB, Christensson K, Matthiesen AS, Winberg J, Uvnas-Moberg K. Gastric suction in healthy newborn infants. Effects on circulation and developing feeding behaviour. Acta Paediatr Scand 1987 July;76(4):566-72.

(9)   Meier PP, Mangurten HH. Breastfeeding the Pre-Term Infant. In: Riordan JM, Auerbach KG, editors. Breastfeeding and Human Lactation.Boston: Jones & Bartlett; 1993. p. 253-78.

(10) Wahlberg V. The "Kangaroo method" and breastfeedng in low birth weight babies. Nytt on U-landshalsovard 1991;5(3):22-7.

(11) Colson S. Biological nurturing. Biological Nurturing 2005.

HOW THE BRAIN DEVELOPS AND WORKS: NEUROSCIENCE

Her brain is the most important part of your baby!

It will make her what she will become.

Early experience makes the brain what it is.

Your baby's brain is wired by you!

The brain is a sensory organ; it collects signals which fire sensitive cells called neurons. As they fire, they wire connections and circuits in the brain.

These circuits need sleep to organize properly.

These pathways develop in layers that make a baby grow emotionally and socially.

In her mother's womb, the baby is already collecting messages or "sensations" of touch, sound, and warmth from her mother. When she is born she is expecting these familiar sounds.

What a shock then to be separated from her mother, and so the baby feels unsafe, and her brain fires and wires for stress and avoidance. Prematures are even more sensitive and struggle even more to find their balance so they need skin-to-skin contact even more than full term babies. She may struggle to connect with people. This poorer social development has long-term effects on health.

We need to do all that we can to protect her brain from harm. We also need to positively help her brain growth to be healthy. We will look at physical health and emotional health

By 28 weeks the fetus has the most nerve cells she will ever have. She will keep the circuits that fire often and lose those that do not fire.

The neurons will move and be coated in myelin fat to speed up the sending of messages in the brain

Being a caring parent is a vital and wonderful "job" for the next few years.

Your baby needs you to do it!

Note: This chapter may seem complicated, but is important to know as it will change the way that you care for your baby practically!

The nerve cells in your baby's brain are expecting certain messages at particular times during development. Your baby is expecting the sound of your voice and heart beat, your smell, and the sight of your face. These will make her feel safe, and protected. She is expecting quiet muffled sounds in her ears and darkness for her developing eyes. These expectations are linked to basic pathways on which later pathways will be built.

To understand your baby's needs it may be helpful to know how her brain has been growing, and why protecting the brain is so important for the <u>quality</u> of her survival.

How the brain grows and develops from conception:

In the first days after conception a tube forms with a swelling at one end which is the beginning of the brain and the spinal cord. In the tube there are neurons (or nerve cells) which collect information and conduct messages. The neurons are tree-shaped, and both branches and roots make a network in the brain, with connections to the body. Some nerves are covered with myelin, a fatty membrane, which speeds up the sending of messages. Myelin comes from special fatty acids only found in breast milk.

<u>Inside mother (gestation)</u>

▸   From 0–14 weeks the genes mostly decide your baby's development. After that, experience and sensations are more important in deciding how the brain grows.

▸   Between 10 to14 weeks the brain appears and the eyes start to develop.

▸   By 20 weeks all brain structures are in place and working!

▸   By 23 weeks the fetus is conscious and aware. Her tiny ears hear and her eyes react to light. She can taste, swallow, and suck her thumb to soothe herself.

▸   By 28 weeks the fetus has the most nerve cells she will ever have. No more are produced after this. (These cells still need to move to their final positions and to branch and connect to other nerve cells). By 28 weeks the brain is developed well enough for the baby to survive outside the womb – on her mother. (The lungs and other organs may need help.)

During the last third of pregnancy development is about connecting the neurons (1).

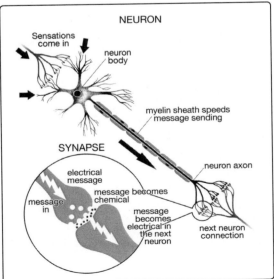

> ## "Cells that fire together, wire together, and those that don't, won't" *Carla Shatz*

Those nerve cells that are not fired-wired, are removed, they are unnecessary and in the way! And so 50% of the nerve cells that the baby had at 28 weeks have disappeared by 40 weeks (2).

> ## "Use it or lose it"

'SAFE' on mum's chest

The nerve cells in your baby's brain are expecting certain messages at particular times during development. Your baby is expecting the sound of your voice and heart beat, your smell, and the sight of your face. These will make her feel safe, and protected. She is expecting quiet muffled sounds in her ears and darkness for her developing eyes. These expectations are linked to basic pathways on which later pathways will be built.

In skin-to-skin contact the baby feels SAFE. The mothers body helps the baby's body to find a physically healthy balance or stability. This sets healthy set points for her heart rate, blood pressure and oxygen saturation. If the baby is later stressed, she will be able to cope better and return to stability or "self-regulate".

The same thing happens with the baby's emotional balance. New neuroscience has shown that the baby's brain translates all sensations into emotions. These help the baby to know what people or situations are good Emotion is core to making any decision. Good is felt as reward which the baby seeks or approaches. Feeling SAFE fires the basic brain pathway to approach (3;4) so the baby will open her eyes, even at a very early gestational age and make eye-to-eye contact with her mother to bond and attach to her. Your baby is conscious and aware and is an emotional being with needs just like yours. Your emotions shape your baby's emotions (7).

When did your baby first open her eyes? ....

The opposite is also true.

A baby separated from her mother will feel UNSAFE. She will cry, her blood pressure and heart rate will increase and she will struggle with her breathing. She will not have help to set healthy physical set points.

On an emotional level separation fires the avoidance pathway in the brain. This baby will look inwards and struggle to cope emotionally, and will avoid eye contact.

Repeating these patterns wires the circuits of the baby's early personality. The ability to decide appropriately to approach or avoid is the foundation for her health and well-being now, and her mental health later (5;6).

> **Your baby's brain is wired by you!**

You, Mum and Dad, need to make sure that your baby's brain is wired for <u>good</u> things, not bad.

> **Being caring parents is a vital and wonderful "job" for the next few years.**
> **Your baby needs you to do it!**

If your baby is born early, these needs for gentle and peaceful safe sensations are not met. For a prem baby, brain development will now be in the busy, noisy NICU, in an incubator, separated from mother. No wonder being born prematurely is such a shock for her! The messages the brain receives are unexpected and frightening. The baby will withdraw, and therefore fire avoidance pathways in the brain.

> **So how can you help your baby's brain to develop properly?**
> **Give your baby skin-to-skin contact**

It is skin-to-skin contact which is the expected and therefore most important sensation after birth. Almost all the healthy sensations are provided on mum's chest. Skin-to-skin contact also stimulates the baby to breastfeed (8). This way all the good sensations are provided!

The baby's brain collects all the sensations together and organizes them to make sense of her world and wires her brain for health and well-being and calmness.

This skin-to-skin holding and breastfeeding is what is feeding your baby's brain.

Which of these facts were new to you?

....

....

....

....

....

Sleep is very important for brain wiring, state organization and memory formation, as we shall see in the next chapter.

> **"The brain is designed to be sculpted into its final configuration by the effects of early experiences." (Martin Teicher) (14)**
> **These experiences depend on a primary caregiver, usually the mother.**

SENSATIONS THAT WIRE THE BRAIN

SEES
Mum's eyes

SMELLS
Mum's milk

TASTES
Mum's milk

Hand TOUCH
Mum's skin

Skin-to-skin
CONTACT

Ear HEARS
Mum's voice

MOVES
with Mum

Back FEELS
Mum's arm
holding

WARMED on
Mum's front

- Eye-to-eye contact with her mother sparks the part of the brain (the amygdala), which helps the baby bond with her mum and grow her emotional intelligence. Face-to-face contact sparks the brain pathways for belonging and social attachment.

- Smell is probably the strongest sense in tiny babies. She smells your breast and breast milk which are familiar and calming. The smell of breast milk sends messages to the stomach to release enzymes to digest the milk (9;10).

- She tastes your milk – exactly what she needs to grow.

- Her hands feel the softness of your skin. Often a mother will hold her baby's tiny hand. Messages reach the mothers brain, to release the hormone oxytocin. This is the love hormone, but it also releases milk and calms mother (11;12).

- The baby's chest feels the skin-to-skin contact which sends messages to the front of the baby's brain to say that she is safe and can relax. This wires her amygdala or emotional brain for health and "approach" behaviour (4).

- Skin-to-skin contact makes baby feel warm and so she feels safe (13).

- Your arm around her back holding and containing her stimulates the part of her brain for deep touch, making her feel that she belongs and that she is loved and safe.

- Mum and baby move together, and this is familiar and reassuring.

- Her ears hear your voice and heartbeat – so familiar and soothing from all her months inside you.

Fine Print Page – How the Brain Develops

1. Carla Shatz studied how vision developed in fetal kittens, she blocked the firing of the neurons, and the kittens were born with perfect eyes, but they were blind.

2. This human study shows the higher number of neurons babies have compared to adults, albeit in a specific area of the brain.

3–5. Amodio describes the BAS (Behavioural Approach System) in detail. The two articles by Schore are an extensive review of this neuroscience, and pages 25 – 33 in "secure attachment" deal with the skin contact and tactile effects on brain pathways, and the subsequent regulation and orientation behaviour.

6. Panksepp's research bridges basic brain neuroscience with psychology and psychiatry, and this book is a detailed treatise of this work in mammals. He says "use it or lose it" (page 17), but also summarises developmental trajectories, contrasting effects of "social comfort" against "separation distress" (page 263).

7. The first half of this book describes how the mother baby interactions and the positive sensory environment shape the baby's brain, its intelligence, and its ability to communicate and speak.

8. In this study, authors show that "Early postpartum mother-baby skin-to-skin contact had a powerful influence (P<0.001) over the duration of exclusive breastfeeding up to 4-6 months and was found to be more significant than early initiation of breastfeeding (P<0.05)." This reflects early influences on brain pathways that make breastfeeding easier. Smell is especially important … as follows:

9–10. Porter has studied olfaction (smell) in the newborn period, and shows how important this is for the newborn. This is important, because we adults have lost the olfactory capacity babies have, and so ignore it. But babies depend on it !!! The sense of security the baby has comes in part from the continuity provided by smells in the uterus (amniotic fluid) to the skin-to-skin contact and then the breasts (milk).

11–12. Kerstin Uvnas-Moberg describes the "love hormone" oxytocin, the book reference (11) is written for a lay reader. 'It seems that tactile, olfactory, visual, and perhaps other types of sensory stimuli contribute to the adaptive changes in both mother and infant. Central oxytocinergic mechanisms activated in connection with birth and breastfeeding seem to be involved in the behavioural changes".

13. This is the introductory article of a hard cover journal, all of which deals with the sensory environment. Quote: "Future NICU design should recognize that the baby must spend most of its time in its mother's arms to get the full benefit of her sensory environment as experienced throughout our evolution."

14. This article refers to the normal brain development described briefly in this chapter, but goes on to describe maladaptive changes that follow from stress and trauma.

Reference List

(1)   Shatz CJ. The developing brain. Sci Am 1992 September;267(3):60-7.

(2)   Abitz M, Nielsen RD, Jones EG, Laursen H, Graem N, Pakkenberg B. Excess of neurons in the human newborn mediodorsal thalamus compared with that of the adult. Cerebral Cortex (New York, N Y : 1991) 2007 November 11;17(11):2573-8.

(3)   Amodio DM, Master SL, Yee CM, Taylor SE. Neurocognitive components of the behavioral inhibition and activation systems: Implications for theories of self-regulation. Psychophysiology 2008;45:11-1.

(4)   Schore AN. Effects of a secure attachment relationship on right brain development, affect regulation, and infant mental health. Infant Mental Health Journal 2001;22(1-2):7-66.

(5)   Schore AN. The effects of early relational trauma on right brain development, affect regulation, and infant mental health. Infant Mental Health Journal 2001;22(1-2):201-69.

(6)   Panksepp J. Affective neuroscience. Oxford Univarsity Press; 1998.

(7)   Greenspan SI, Shanker SG, Phil D. The First Idea: How symbols, language, and intelligence evolved from our primate ancestors to modern humans. 1st ed. Cambridge: Da Capo Press; 2006.

(8)   Vaidya K, Sharma A, Dhungel S. Effect of early mother-baby close contact over the duration of exclusive breastfeeding. Nepal Medical College Journal: NMCJ 2005 December;7(2):138-40.

(9)   Porter RH, Winberg J. Unique salience of maternal breast odors for newborn infants. Neurosci Biobehav Rev 1999;23(3):439-49.

(10) Porter RH. The biological significance of skin-to-skin contact and maternal odours. Acta Paediatrica 2004 December;93(12):1560-2.

(11) Uvnas-Moberg K, Francis R. The oxytocin factor: tapping the hormome of calm, love, and healing. MA Da Capo Press 2003;(Chapter 8 Nursing):93-103.

(12) Uvnas-Moberg K. Neuroendocrinology of the mother-child interaction. Trends In Endocrinology And Metabolism: TEM 1996 May;7(4):126-31.

(13) White RD. Mothers' arms--the past and future locus of neonatal care? Clin Perinatol 2004 June;31(2):383-7, ix.

(14) Teicher MH, Andersen SL, Polcari A, Anderson CM, Navalta CP. Developmental neurobiology of childhood stress and trauma. Psychiatr Clin North Am 2002 June;25(2):397-426.

PROTECT SLEEP

All babies need to sleep a lot.

Premature babies need to sleep even more

A prem baby in an incubator does not sleep properly.

A baby in skin-to-skin contact will sleep better as she feels SAFE.

On your chest she will have the right temperature, and be hearing your heart beat, her head will be covered to shut out bright lights and to muffle sound. Her brain will have the chance to organize and form healthy pathways.

Babies' brains need sleep for memory formation and completing brain circuits.

Babies need to sleep and wake in cycles to get the best brain wiring. Good sleep cycling only happens when a baby is with her mother.

When a baby is sleeping she can use all her food energy for growing.

Do NOT wake her from quiet sleep.

Protect your baby's sleep and you will help her brain development.

All babies need to sleep to sort out the wiring of their brains.

Let us look at <u>what is happening inside the mother</u>. Before baby is born she sleeps a lot. In your womb, your baby has touch and contact, gentle movement and muffled sounds; your baby's brain collects these gentle messages and stores them. She follows her mother's day-night rhythm, but she also has her own sleep – wake cycles. Babies have two kinds of sleep states.

The first stage is called "rapid-eye-movement sleep", or REM sleep. The baby is actually asleep, but the brain is very active and the eyes move under the eyelids. In her mother's womb, the baby's brain is firing to start making organized pathways (1;2). This happens without stimulations from the outside that normally make nerve cells fire. Inside the mother the baby's brain is not over-stimulated. The brain has time to organize all of the pathways that are being fired (3).

After REM or active sleep, the baby needs a time of quiet sleep. This is called "non-REM 4" (or NR4 in diagram). It can be recognized by a very regular heart beat. During this time the brain pathways are completed and secured (4). After that, her brain is ready for another set of messages.

Another period of REM sleep follows. If the baby is going to wake, it will be during or after REM sleep. The cycling of REM and non-REM sleep is very important for growth and brain wiring.

When the <u>prem is born too early</u>, she is placed in a NICU with bright lights, lots of noise, distractions and many people. This is an overload of messages. The prem in an incubator does not sleep-cycle properly, and so can not sort out all these messages. Because her sleep is disturbed, her memory formation and brain wiring are disorganised. She is alone and separated from her mother so she often cries until she is too exhausted. When she eventually does sleep, she may sink into a deep apnoea sleep, where she is so tired that she can even forget to breathe.

SLEEP CYCLING
Separation vs Skin-to-Skin

Incubator   **SSC**

Chaotic behaviour pattern, little sleep | Regular sleep cycling

To <u>help your prem sleep</u> and brain wire properly, return her as closely as possible to the womb environment or what she had inside you (5). Holding your baby in skin-to-skin contact on your chest will help her to feel peaceful, and have sleep and wake cycling to control her state properly and so help healthy brain development (6;7).

When the baby is awake, or in REM sleep, she is collecting messages which go to the surface of the brain (cortex). At 27–30 weeks the prem baby is only alert for very short times. When she goes into quiet sleep (non-REM) the information is sent to the emotional centre of the brain (called the amygdala). Every physical sensation is stored with an emotion in the brain. When the baby starts to wake up, early REM sleep sends these messages to the front of the brain, which makes the

SLEEP WIRES BRAIN PATHWAYS

1. Messages are collected in cortex
2. In non-REM sleep messages moved to emotional brain (amygdala)
3. End of sleep cycle, messages to front of brain (approach/ avoid)
4. Organized brain circuit now complete

decision to approach or avoid. This organized circuit of pathways is like a drawer system in which the memory is stored (8).

It is possible for you to learn how to tell which state your baby is in. When she is awake, her eyes are open and she is moving her arms and legs. She will then become drowsy and slow down. There may be small twitches of her fingers and face muscles. The distinctive "rapid eye movement" is not always easy to see. Her breathing and heart rate are a bit irregular. Watch your baby for the small signs that tell you what state she is in, so that you know what the best care at that time will be.

> **When she is in quiet sleep, her breathing is very even, and her body is very still and calm.**

In quiet sleep she has a normal heart rate and her temperature tends to be more even than when she is awake. It is important not to disturb her at this time as she is sleeping quietly and is in an "organised" or unstressed state.

What a baby does and how she reacts depends on her state of being asleep or awake. The ability to control awake and asleep is called state organization. One of the main problems for a prem separated from her mother is that she has bad "state organization". In the diagram you can see how incubator babies swing chaotically from one extreme to the other. Crying is stressful and wastes calories; there is also a risk of bleeding in the brain. In deep sleep there is a risk of apnoea. In skin-to-skin contact, the mother's body settles and calms the baby. Your baby's state cycles from good quality sleep to waking and feeding.

Remember, good sleep cycling is vital for brain wiring and this only happens with mother. For the prem, quiet sleep is even more essential, as the brain is more sensitive.

Mum and baby also get into a rhythm of sleeping at the same time, ("sleep synchrony") (9).

The mum and baby act as "co-regulators" (10).

Your baby can be woken after REM sleep, but NOT during quiet sleep.
Protect your baby's sleep and you will help her brain development

Prem babies sleep a lot and may need to be woken for feeding after a quiet sleep period. Small feeds every 60–90 minutes are better as they match the sleep cycle. Hold your baby in skin-to-skin contact on your chest at least a full hour after a feed so that she can complete a full sleep-wake cycle, as well as absorb all of her food properly.

Many books on baby care say the baby should sleep 2–4 hours at a time. "Popular belief" at present says the baby should be "trained to sleep". In the first few months this does not apply.

Fine Print Page – Protect Sleep

1–2. These are both rather complex papers, but describe in detail what REM is and what it does. There is some controversy as always, but the need for REM and NREM sleep is undisputed.

3. This article summarises sleep development more practically, and covers most of the content of this chapter. Quote: "REM and NREM sleep cycling are essential for early neurosensory development, learning and memory, and preservation of brain plasticity for the life of the individual."

4. Sleep has been studied extensively, but there are fewer studies looking at the effect of skin-to-skin contact on sleep. This paper concludes "The patterns demonstrated by the SSC group are analogous to more mature sleep organization. SSC may be used as an intervention to improve sleep organization in this population of preterm infants.".

5. This study looked specifically at premature infants, confirming " … a significant increase in sleep time for the neonates during skin-to-skin contact (with) less agitation, apnea, and bradycardia episodes and maintained stable oxygen saturation … safe even for very small neonates and is well tolerated".

6. Feldman has published a number of follow-up studies, and in this shows that after SSC, prems at birth have "more mature state distribution and more organized sleep-wake cyclicity".

7. This paper explains state organization, and also shows that full term babies sleep better when in skin-to-skin contact.

8. Another complex paper… but describes in great detail how sleep cycling works… the hippocampus is studied here, and is closely linked to the amygdala.

9. Sleep synchrony is also part of the contentious "co-sleeping debate"! It is safer for mother and baby to sleep together, but co-sleeping must also be done in a safe manner. (http://www.nd.edu/~jmckenn1/lab/faq.html)

10. In animal studies, "mutual care giving between newborn and mothers" is described; Gene Cranston Anderson was perhaps the first to describe this in humans!

Reference List

(1) Marks GA, Shaffery JP, Oksenberg A, Speciale SG, Roffwarg HP. A functional role for REM sleep in brain maturation. Behavioural Brain Research 1995 July;69(1-2):1-11.

(2) Mirmiran M. The function of fetal/neonatal rapid eye movement sleep. Behavioural Brain Research 1995 July;69(1-2):13-22.

(3) Graven S. Sleep and Brain Development. Clinics in Perinatology 2006;33:693-706.

(4) Ludington-Hoe SM, Johnson MW, Morgan K, Lewis T, Gutman J, Wilson PD et al. Neurophysiologic Assessment of Neonatal Sleep Organization: Preliminary Results of a Randomized, Controlled Trial of Skin Contact With Preterm Infants. Journal of the American Academy of Child & Adolescent Psychiatry 2006 December;45(12):1455.

(5) Messmer PR, Rodriguez S, Adams J, Wells-Gentry J, Washburn K, Zabaleta I et al. Effect of kangaroo care on sleep time for neonates. Pediatr Nurs 1997 July;23(4):408-14.

(6) Feldman R, Weller A, Sirota L, Eidelman AI. Skin-to-Skin contact (Kangaroo care) promotes self-regulation in premature infants: sleep-wake cyclicity, arousal modulation, and sustained exploration. Dev Psychol 2002 March;38(2):194-207.

(7) Ferber SG, Makhoul IR. The effect of skin-to-skin contact (kangaroo care) shortly after birth on the neurobehavioral responses of the term newborn: a randomized, controlled trial. Pediatrics 2004 April;113(4):858-65.

(8) Ji D, Wilson MA. Coordinated memory replay in the visual cortex and hippocampus during sleep. Nature Neuroscience 2007;10(1):100-7.

(9) McKenna JJ, Mosko SS. Sleep and arousal, synchrony and independence, among mothers and infants sleeping apart and together (same bed): an experiment in evolutionary medicine. Acta Paediatr Suppl 1994 June;397:94-102.

(10) Anderson GC. Risk in mother-infant separation postbirth. Image: Journal of Nursing Scholarship 1989;21(4):196-9.

SEPARATION AND STRESS

> **Being separated from mother is stressful for all babies.**

Your baby's security, her SAFE place is you, her mother. She will protest by crying if she is separated from you.

When a baby cries her heart rate and blood pressure go up, and oxygen saturation goes down.

> **If a premature cries she is at increased risk for a brain bleed.**

If she cries for too long your baby may go into despair behaviour.

When babies are in the wrong place, separated from mother, they have defensive behaviours which may cause changes to brain wiring that are harmful in the future.

> **The premature baby is not in an incubator because she is unstable, She is unstable because she is in an incubator!** *N. Bergman 2004*

Babies should not need to cry.

Prem babies should never cry.

Severe stress without a parent to support her is toxic to the newborn's brain.

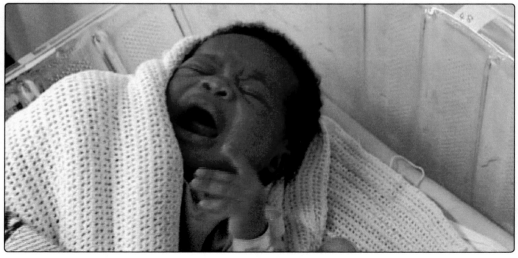

Protest:

When a baby is separated from her mother, her safe place, her response is often to cry. Crying is the baby's way of communicating with her Mum to pick her up (1), feed her, soothe her or change her nappy. Crying is also her protest that she is alone and frightened. Her arms and legs move to get Mum's attention (2).

Hard crying also forces open a valve between the two parts of the heart, so that blood without oxygen is sent to the brain instead of the lungs (3). It is dangerous for the brain to be without oxygen.

The prem's brain feels unsafe and releases stress hormones like cortisol which increase her heart rate, blood pressure and speeds up her breathing. If you imagine the blood vessels carrying blood from the heart to the brain, they are like a tree trunk. These vessels make thinner branches and eventually tiny twigs. When the baby cries a lot, the blood pressure and volume increases too much in these tiny vessels. They may burst causing a bleed in the "ventricles", which are spaces in the middle of the brain where spinal fluid is made (4).

Stress will be seen in the baby's body as it makes her back arch and her legs and arms move a lot. This uses up a lot of energy which the baby should be using to grow.

Stress will release the hormone somatostatin which inhibits growth hormone and prevents the stomach from absorbing food effectively (5).

> **Stress will affect the emotions and mind of the baby; as she will think that "nobody hears me crying or cares that I am alone and frightened". In the brain, there is "hyper-arousal" or vigilance (6).**

Despair:

If the baby cries for a long time, she becomes exhausted, runs out of calories and may have a headache; because of that she stops crying. At this stage, <u>despair</u> sets in. It is a more dangerous stage of the defence programme. In this time, the stress hormones are still circulating, trying to speed the body up (for a "fight or flight" reaction to danger). But at the same time her brain sends nerve signals to slow the body down to save energy. The baby's body does not know how to cope with these opposite messages (7)!

Her heart rate slows by ten beats per minute and her temperature goes down by 1°C to conserve energy for as long as possible in the hope that her mother will come back. Her breathing may become irregular, she moves less and her body is still. Do not think that this baby in the incubator is resting or sleeping. She has gone into a state called "dissociation" or despair.

The baby feels abandoned and withdraws into herself. Research has shown that these babies have increased activity in the avoidance centre of the brain. When

"AM I SAFE ?"

PLACE CHOICE EFFECT RESULT

MOTHER "APPROACH" BREAST- BONDING
"Safe" ➡(Calming) ➡ FEEDING➡ GROWTH

OTHER ➡"AVOID" ➡ PROTEST➡VIGILANCE
"Unsafe" (Stressful) DESPAIR SURVIVAL

this happens a lot, her brain-wiring will make her distrust people and be emotionally distant; she will have trouble bonding (8).

A tiny baby has not yet developed a separate sense of self. Her very being is tied up with her mother for the first months of life. When a tiny baby is separated from her mother she goes through what psychologists call "annihilation anxiety", she fears that she does not exist, or that she will die (9).

This is why a baby reacts so strongly to being separated from her mother.

> **A baby needs to be held by her mother for physical and emotional well-being.**

For a premature baby this separation is even more frightening. The prem should be developing and maturing in the womb, "a designer milieu". Instead, she suddenly finds herself in a noisy NICU with bright lights and the sharp noises of beeping machines. Worst of all, she is separated from her mother! Imagine what this does to her developing brain! It causes long term physical and emotional problems. This tiny brain is now brain-wiring for a life that it expects to be stressful (10). The defence pathways become this baby's way of coping with stress instead of calmer thinking and trusting. In this situation, the baby is wary and alert and at risk for developing high blood pressure later in life (11). Not having food when she is hungry makes her body store food more and she will tend to obesity and diabetes when she is grown up. (8;12)

All of the above sounds horrible! But it is new evidence, feel free to look up the reference on the fine print page.

How can you tell if you baby is in protest or despair? Your baby will show small signs that say "stop" or "give me a break or help me to calm down". Learn to recognize the specific signs of your own baby being "disorganised".

Sitting on air (protest)
Arms extended

Looking away
(gaze aversion)

Stop sign (protest)

> **Watch your own baby carefully and respond to her messages.**

Hiding face (despair)

Yawning (despair)

These are some of the signs of a baby who is stressed and disorganised:

Put a tick next to which signs you have seen when your baby is upset.

Protest

▸ She cries.
▸ She holds her breath – apnoea.
▸ Her heart rate increases.
▸ Her blood pressure increases.
▸ Her skin colour becomes red, darkens or becomes blotchy.
▸ She extends or stretches her arms and legs out sideways.
▸ She arches her back stiffly.
▸ She spreads her arms out wide and holds them stiffly.
▸ She splays her fingers and toes.
▸ She puts her hands in front of her face with a 'stop sign'.
▸ Her movements are jerky and there are twitches or tremors.
▸ She "sits on air" with her legs up in the air at right angles to her body.
▸ She fusses and squirms.
▸ She sneezes, hiccups and spits up.

Despair

▸ Her breathing is irregular.
▸ Her heart rate decreases.
▸ Her oxygen saturation decreases.
▸ She looks away from you.
▸ She becomes limp.
▸ She yawns.
▸ She frowns.
▸ Small twitches of face muscles and fingers.

How to calm a distressed baby

If your prem is doing any of these things she is in distress and needs you! Ideally, she wants to be picked up and held in skin-to-skin contact. For ANY baby you can gently place your hand over her body and hold your hand still. You can also cup one hand around her head and one around her feet to contain her. Flex her legs and bring her hand or fist next to her mouth. This will give her security. Help your baby to find ways to keep herself calm. This is called "self-soothing" or "self-regulating".

Do **not** rock her or shake or jig her up and down or pat her back.

The next chapter on developmental care will give you more ideas on how to avoid stress for your baby.

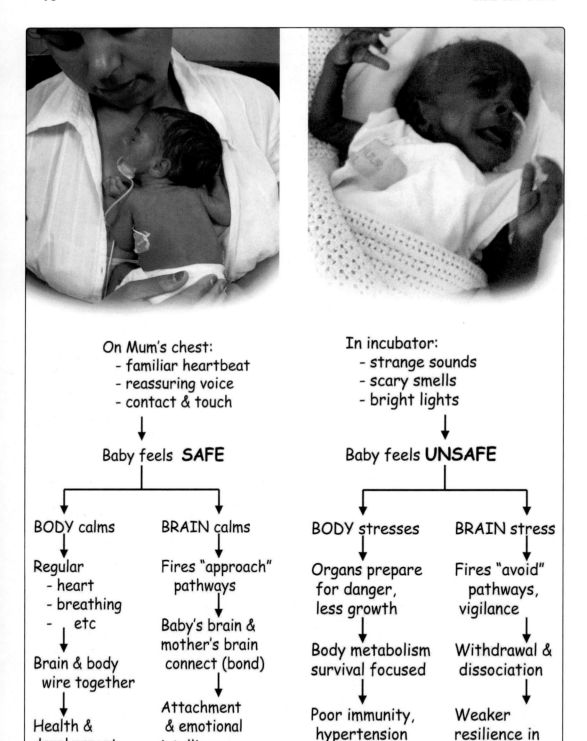

On Mum's chest:
- familiar heartbeat
- reassuring voice
- contact & touch

↓

Baby feels **SAFE**

BODY calms	BRAIN calms
↓	↓
Regular - heart - breathing - etc	Fires "approach" pathways
↓	↓
Brain & body wire together	Baby's brain & mother's brain connect (bond)
↓	↓
Health & development	Attachment & emotional intelligence

In incubator:
- strange sounds
- scary smells
- bright lights

↓

Baby feels **UNSAFE**

BODY stresses	BRAIN stress
↓	↓
Organs prepare for danger, less growth	Fires "avoid" pathways, vigilance
↓	↓
Body metabolism survival focused	Withdrawal & dissociation
↓	↓
Poor immunity, hypertension diabetes later	Weaker resilience in later life

Fine Print Page – Separation and Stress

1. Separation distress calls are universal among mammals, including humans! Quote: "this cry is not dependent on earlier social experience and may be a genetically encoded reaction to separation".

2. This article describes the actual brain circuits in the parents that are activated by the above distress call, quote: "networks of highly conserved hypothalamic-midbrain-limbic-paralimbic-cortical circuits act in concert to support aspects of parent response to infants". These make parents "generally compelled to approach a crying infant … Infant cry–care loops may thus be thought of as part of an elaborate, dynamic and interactive communication system that maintains proximity to and elicits care from caregivers".

3. Summarises many adverse effects, and identifies skin-to-skin contact as effective care!

4. This is an old, but original study that showed effect of crying, opening the foramen ovale, with right to left shunting, as seen in the fetus.

5. Somatostatin "lowers the rate of gastric emptying, reduces smooth muscle contractions and blood flow within the intestine. Collectively, has the overall effect of decreasing the rate of nutrient absorption." http://www.vivo.colostate.edu/hbooks/pathphys/endocrine/otherendo/somatostatin.html

6. Perry describes responses to threat, the first of which is vigilance, then freeze, finally dissociation.

7. Schore describes these in slightly different terms, (hyperarousal), with detail on the neuroanatomy. Quote: "...rapid alterations of ANS sympathetic ergotropic hyperarousal and parasympathetic trophotropic hypoarousal create chaotic biochemical alterations, a toxic neurochemistry in the developing brain."

8. Teicher describes the neuronal and anatomical changes that abuse and neglect makes in the brain, but importantly suggests that these are adaptations to make the brain cope better in harsh world. But this adaptation is actually "maladaptive" in the social arena.

9. Hofer shows that early experiences do in fact impact on the quality of attachment. Quote: "behavioral, physiological and neural processes underlie the psychological constructs of attachment theory. It has become apparent that the unique features of early infant attachment reflect certain unique features of early infant sensory and motor integration, early learning, communication, motivation and the regulation of biobehavioral systems by the mother–infant interaction."

10. Pain is one of the main experiences of prems, and Anand describes some known consequences. Quote: "Perinatal brain plasticity increases the vulnerability to early adverse experiences, thus leading to abnormal development and behavior."

11. This book describes the latest research field: epigenetics, whereby we now have clearer understanding of the mechanisms of how environment and experience change the brain and the body.

12. Barker was the first to identify such effects, looking at babies born with low-birth weight. He described a "thrifty phenotype" with altered metabolism leading to obesity and hypertension, and later diabetes.

Reference List

(1) Christensson K, Cabrera T, Christensson E, Uvnas-Moberg K, Winberg J. Separation distress call in the human neonate in the absence of maternal body contact. Acta Paediatr 1995 May;84(5):468-73.

(2) Swain JE, Lorberbaum JP, Kose S, Strathearn L. Brain basis of early parent-infant interactions: psychology, physiology, and in vivo functional neuroimaging studies. Journal of Child Psychology & Psychiatry 2007 March;48(3/4):262-87.

(3) Ludington-Hoe SM, Cong X, Hashemi F. Infant crying: nature, physiologic consequences, and select interventions. Neonatal Network: NN 2002 March;21(2):29-36.

(4) Lind J. Changes in the circulation and lungs at birth. Acta Paediatrica Supplementum 1960 March;49 (Suppl 122):39-52.

(5) Widstrom AM, Marchini G, Matthiesen AS, Werner S, Winberg J, Uvnas-Moberg K. Nonnutritive sucking in tube-fed preterm infants: effects on gastric motility and gastric contents of somatostatin. J Pediatr Gastroenterol Nutr 1988 July;7(4):517-23.

(6) Perry BD, Pollard RA, Blakely TL, Baker WL, Vigilante D. Childhood trauma, the neurobiology of adaptation and "use-dependent" development of the brain. How"states" become "traits". Infant Mental health 1995;16(4):271-91.

(7) Schore AN. The effects of early relational trauma on right brain development, affect regulation, and infant mental health. Infant Mental Health Journal 2001;22(1-2):201-69.

(8) Teicher MH, Andersen SL, Polcari A, Anderson CM, Navalta CP. Developmental neurobiology of childhood stress and trauma. Psychiatr Clin North Am 2002 June;25(2):397-426.

(9) Hofer MA. The psychobiology of early attachment. Clinical Neuroscience Research 2005;XX:1-10.

(10) Anand KJ, Scalzo FM. Can adverse neonatal experiences alter brain development and subsequent behavior? Biology Of The Neonate 2000 February;77(2):69-82.

(11) Gluckman P, Hanson M. The Fetal Matrix Evolution, Development and Disease. The Press Syndicate of the University of Cambridge; 2005.

(12) Barker DJ. In utero programming of chronic disease. Clinical Science (London, England: 1979) 1998 August;95(2):115-28.

DEVELOPMENTAL CARE

> **Things you do now for your prem can make a huge difference later.**

You, her parents, are her SAFE place! BE THERE! GET INVOLVED!

> **Prems are very small and very sensitive; they sense everything!**

Protect your baby's senses.

The best developmental care – on mum.

- ▶ <u>Touch</u>: skin-to-skin contact should start from birth, or as soon as possible. Hold your baby firmly, close, still and contained she will be calmer to grow faster. Handle her gently; flex her legs and arms with her hands near her mouth.
- ▶ <u>Smell</u>: your baby longs for the smell of your breast and your breast milk; avoid strongly perfumed soap.
- ▶ <u>Taste</u>: your baby should taste your breast milk.
- ▶ <u>Sound</u>: your prem knows your voice, speak to her!
- ▶ <u>Sight</u>: your baby can recognize your face.

Respond as soon as she shows signs of discomfort and before her body has becomes severely stressed or sick.

> **WATCH YOUR INDIVIDUAL BABY AND LEARN WHAT UPSETS HER.**
> **Fix or change what you can.**

Nest and position her in the incubator to support her developing muscles.

Your prem is aware and has feelings. Talk to her as a person and tell her what you are going to do. She must never be treated like an object.

Modern technology can keep smaller and younger babies alive, but we want these babies to have the best <u>quality</u> of life as well, so we have to treat them extra gently. Her brain needs to be protected from stress as it is very fragile.

"Developmental Care" is a term used by many people and can mean many different things. Here I am using the term Developmental Care to mean a gentle method of caring for all babies, especially for the premature baby, which will support the healthy development of body, brain and emotions by minimizing stress, and so reducing problems for the baby in the future.

Mum and Dad, your prem baby was expecting another few weeks of being held curled up, warm, quiet, safe and protected, and being fed continuously in the womb. Now she has been born early, and lies in a noisy, busy, bright NICU. What a shock these changes must be for her!! No wonder she is frightened, cries and is unstable!

As you can see from the table below, holding your baby in skin-to-skin contact makes her feel as if she is back in the womb and restores her to her safe place!

In Mum's womb baby expects	In incubator, baby experiences	On Mum's chest in skin-to-skin
Arms bent	Arms stick out sideways	Arms bent
Legs bent or flexed	Legs often extended	Legs bent or flexed
Quiet and peaceful sounds	Noisy, busy NICU, alarms	Quiet and peaceful sounds
Mum's womb contains her	No containment, no boundaries	Mum's arms contain her
Back curled	Lies flat on back	Back curled
Fed continuously	Fed 2-4 hourly	Fed frequently
Nearly dark in womb	Bright lights	Gentle light inside shirt
Feels SAFE	Feels unsafe / frightened and alone	Feels SAFE
Mum's womb holds her	Handled by many nurses & doctors	Mum's arms hold her

Up to now, developmental care has been something that nurses in a NICU do to a baby in an incubator. But as the major stress for tiny babies is to be separated from mother, a prem separated from her mother often struggles to stabilize herself or "self-regulate". Without YOU, your baby cannot keep her stress levels down.

I want to encourage you, <u>MUM</u>, to be with your baby, and to be aware of things that you can do to help your baby to regulate and be stable. You can support her so that she does not feel overwhelmed. She needs skin-to-skin contact to help her physically; to keep her heart rate, breathing, blood pressure and temperature stable. She also needs skin-to-skin contact to calm her down emotionally. (1)

It is mostly accepted that the NICU is not normal, but it is assumed that it is necessary for survival. Now that we know that it can do harm to the developing brain of the premature, we need to think differently.

Placing the prem baby in skin-to-skin contact on mothers chest is the single most cost-effective "developmental care" change that we need to make in modern NICU's. Developmental care does not need to cost a lot of money.

> **Our challenge will be to take the best of modern technology available to a prem and add it in the right place, on mother's chest.**

A picture of Developmental Care could be like looking at ripples in a pond. The very inside circle means giving the best care by handling each individual baby gently to support her own body systems to self-regulate. Physically this means stabilizing her heart rate, breathing, blood pressure and temperature. Emotionally this is seen as being calmer and unstressed The next ripple would be looking how we can make her most comfortable, on mother or in an incubator, so we look at her bed or nest. Then we look at her incubator, then into the larger external NICU ward environment by reducing noise and light to reduce stress, save her energy and help her grow. As she leaves the NICU she will still be small and sensitive and need "Developmental Care" awareness relating to her room and your home. As she grows stronger she will move out into wider society.

Some hospitals work with NIDCAP (Neonatal Individualized Developmental Care and Assessment Programme). This is an advanced, structured developmental care programme. NIDCAP carefully watches how each baby copes, and recommends detailed improvements in care (2;3).

A recent article shows that babies cared for in this way (NIDCAP) recover more quickly. They have less chronic lung disease; they need less ventilation, less CPAP and less extra oxygen. They also go home sooner. It is also cost-effective as hospital stays are shorter. The babies have higher brain development scores at 9 and 12 months. At 18 months' adjusted age, they have less disability, especially less mental delay (10% compared to 30%) (4).

What can you do to help your premature baby?

You, Mum and dad, will want to work to achieve best possible development for your baby. We may never know fully how the brain works and heals, but at least we can say that we did the best possible at the time.

> **Restore the womb environment as far as possible.**

Now, parents and medical personnel can work together to help prems to survive with a better quality of life, physically and emotionally. For the doctor or nurse working in a NICU this will be their full time job, but they change duties every 8 or 12 hours. You are your prem baby's Mum and Dad, and you are the only possible constant support she has. Your touch, your smell, your voices and faces are most important for your baby. The small things that you do now can have a hugely positive impact on your baby's long term development. Understanding the biology behind the development is important. For each sense I will give ideas of what you can do if your baby is in the incubator.

What you can do to help your prem will depend on where she is.

▷   Is she in labour ward?
▷   Is she in the NICU?
▷   How long has she been in NICU?
▷   Does the NICU insist on using incubators?
▷   Is she in a high tech, well-resourced hospital?
▷   Is she in a low tech clinic?

▶ Is a nurse or midwife is with her, or is a doctor deciding on care?

▶ What are the hospital policies on breastfeeding, skin-to-skin contact, etc?

Every NICU is different; there will be parts of the NICU that are wonderful. Appreciate those and encourage the staff members. There will also be some things with which you will disagree now that you know the neuroscience.

Ten years ago, incubator care was standard care for premature babies. This is changing! There is no science proving the safety of incubators, but there is science showing the benefits of baby being on her mum's chest. Every hospital strives to provide ideal care for their patients within their understanding, but they need a specific focus of best care for brain growth, not just for physical survival. The key is skin-to-skin contact. Here, all the developmental care essentials come together, as the baby feels safe. There are no stress hormones; she does not waste energy and can grow faster. She is held securely, and contained; she moves with mum, as she has done in the womb. Her physical development can be good and now you can add mental, emotional and social development!

All this works together to make secure attachment (1).

As we discussed in the neuroscience chapter, <u>it is sensations which fire and wire</u> the brain. You want to give your baby the expected and familiar sensations that are going to

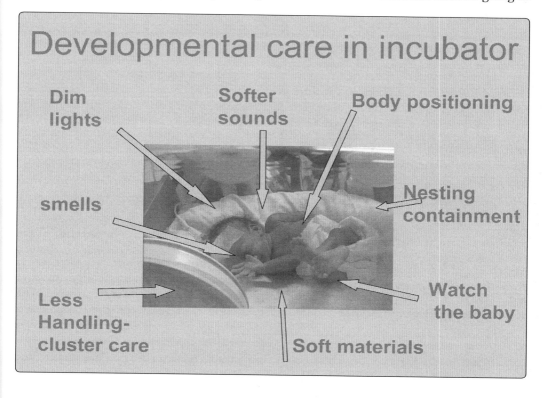

Developmental care in incubator

Dim lights

Softer sounds

Body positioning

smells

Nesting containment

Less Handling- cluster care

Soft materials

Watch the baby

make her feel safe. This feeling of being safe determines how your baby behaves. If she feels safe she will grow well.

Separation from you makes her stressed and you want to avoid stress.

> **Being on your chest in skin-to-skin contact will make your baby feel safe.**

We will look at each sensation in detail:

Touch (this includes, touching, holding, contact, carrying and moving your baby).

The sense of touch develops early inside the mother. The baby inside you has constant pressure from the amniotic fluid.

There are two pathways for touch – deep physical contact or "containment" and light (feather) touch.

Deep physical contact or "containment" is continued contact and pressure on the body. When you hold your baby in skin-to-skin contact (SSC) firmly, close and still, you calm your baby and reassure her that she is safe. This is essential for your tiny prem. Her brain development can continue closer to normal and SSC helps her to develop good muscle tone. Carrying your prem tied on your chest in skin-to-skin contact with her airway stabilized is the best for your prem. Her legs should be flexed and her hands should be near her mouth so that she can comfort herself.

When you need to move her, do so slowly.

Light touch or stroking the skin with feather touch irritates your prem as she is unable to screen out all the messages that she receives. Prems are fragile and do not like to be stroked lightly. (Few adults like to have a spider crawling on them, but everyone needs a firm hug!)

Your baby's skin is very thin and sensitive; remember to use soft natural fibres with a close weave and avoid rough towels.

Contain her arms and legs and hold her still.

Touching your baby if she is in the incubator

Your hospital might be unsure about letting you touch your baby in the incubator. You

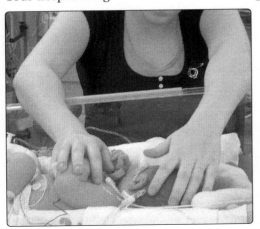

as parents have every right to request this, and modern care understands that it is important. If you or they are worried, leave the monitors on, and watch her stabilize as you place your hands over her. Human touch is essential for your baby.

Your prem in the NICU will be handled by very many nurses and doctors, maybe too many people, often with painful injections or putting tubes down her throat, etc. Mum and Dad, do try to be there to calm your baby when she is becoming stressed. The parents should be the primary care-givers, and nurses should be there to teach and support the parents.

Wash your hands for 2 minutes with unperfumed soap before every contact with your infant. Start by placing your hands firmly and gently over her body. This will help her feel contained and safe. Hold your hands still. It can also be helpful to cup one hand around the top of her head and one hand around her feet or bottom.

Ask the nurses to teach you how to move your baby. Place your hands over her body and hold her legs and arms close to her body so that her body is moved as a whole without her arms flopping out sideways. This will help her vestibular system, which is important for balance.

You can also try putting your little finger in her palm. She may well grasp it. This is her lifeline to help pull her through these long weeks. From 35 weeks onwards, Infant Massage can help.

Nesting and positioning

In your womb, your baby had firm, soft and flexible boundaries. She was curled up in the "fetal position" with her legs together and flexed, and with her arms bent and her hands near her mouth. She has probably been sucking her thumb for a long time as this is self-soothing.

When your baby is born prematurely, the ideal is to restore her to the same fetal position.

> **Hold her in a fetal position with her legs and arms curled up.**

If your baby has to stay in the incubator she is often not strong enough to make herself comfortable and she lies with her legs and arms "extended" or stretched out and often "floppy". It is important to position and flex her by making a tight nest with firm, soft, flexible boundaries with rolls of cloth so that she can lie curled up in the fetal position

Place your hands over her & hold still. Contain her arms & legs.

Bend legs & give feet a boundary to press against.

Cup hands around her head, contain arm, let her hold your finger.

Moving of prem. Hand over body to contain her. Pause if she shows signs of stress.

Make a tight nest to contain her.

> **Nesting and Positioning**

in the incubator. This flexed position helps her to feel secure and contained. The nest should curl her shoulders forward; keep her arms near the midline and her hips to the centre. Help her lie on her side, and sometimes on her tummy. Your baby will need a close boundary to push her feet against.

Over time, positioning affects your baby's development. A prem often lies in an incubator for 6–10 weeks and long-term damage can be done which will cause her problems later on. This can be avoided by correct positioning in the NICU. (See the long-term benefits chapter)

Your prem has very soft bones and should have been developing in the amniotic fluid inside the womb where she would be less affected by gravity. As she has not finished developing, her head can easily become flattened if she lies on her back all the time. By moving your baby's head position even a little bit so that she lies on all sides of the head, her head will stay more rounded. If she stays in the same position for long periods, flat on her back in NICU, she becomes stiff in the shoulders and hips which may cause problems later.

Warmth

When your baby is held in skin-to-skin contact, she will have a much more even temperature than if she were in an incubator.

Mother's skin has a comforting constant temperature. An incubator heats at one time and cools at another so the temperature is always changing.

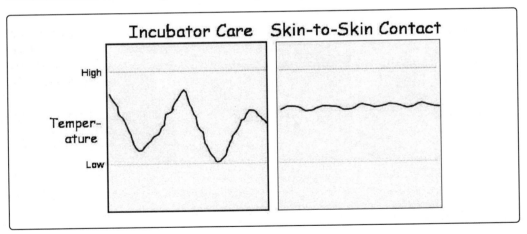

Smell

Smell is one of the strongest senses at birth so she can find the breast and feed to survive.

Your smell will be familiar to her from the amniotic fluid, so she will be reassured and calm. Smelling your breast will encourage early breastfeeding. One of the many benefits of skin-to-skin contact is that normal stomach hormones are released. Her stomach works better, absorbing all the food and this helps her to grow faster. Avoid wearing strong deodorants or perfume. Shower daily and wash your hands regularly (5).

If she is in the incubator some hospitals will insist on alcohol gel, or other antiseptics for your hands. These smell unpleasant to a prem. Wait until they evaporate before touching your baby.

If you are not allowed to hold her, ask if you can take a small soft facecloth or a piece of soft cotton and sleep with it, and then bring it into her incubator. That way she can smell you even when you are not there and this will soothe her (5;6).

Taste

> **Your baby is expecting to taste your breast milk.**

We have looked at how breast milk has the RIGHT and essential nutrients for growth, and how it varies in a wonderful way to give the prem exactly what she needs for completing her development. But taste as a sensation is important for its brain wiring effects, not just for body growth.

Suckling gives your baby a sensation of the nipple and the breast itself. This sensation relaxes your baby; it pulls the nipple onto the top of the mouth (upper palate). This is a soothing centre, and releases hormones for digestion. Sucking on a pacifier can cause many problems with teeth growth and speech later. Even so, a pacifier might be better than leaving a baby to cry!

If your prem is in an incubator, she should still be given your breast milk.

Sound

Inside you, your baby was already hearing by 23 weeks gestational age. The ear sends messages to the brain. Sounds can all be heard, but they are all dampened by mum's body. She can already recognize Mum's and Dad's voices. Sound is tied to day/night rhythms and movement. From 30 weeks onwards, babies like quiet voices with changing rhythms (7).

> **Your baby cannot shut her ears to loud sounds and feels them as pain.**

When she is born, keep noise levels low. Newborns listen simultaneously to everything and cannot screen out sounds. You will learn to pick up your child's individual sensitivity. She will react to some sounds badly and not to others.

Your voice can calm your baby when nothing else can. She has known it and felt safe with it for many months already (8)!

Hearing is what steers the eyes and movement. This means that the ear signal gets attention and the muscle system turns the head and the eyes towards the sound.

If your baby is in an incubator and you are feeling helpless sitting next to her, talk, read and sing to her. Your voice will calm her.

The entire incubator box can become a resonance chamber which magnifies sound.

> **Do not put anything on top of the incubator! Close incubator doors slowly and quietly.**

The NICU should be kept very quiet. Some NICUs have a sound meter to remind people to keep the noise levels low. Cell phones should be switched off and voices kept quiet. Simply dimming the lights encourages people to speak more quietly.

> **Your premature baby's eyes are very sensitive to light. Keep lights dim.**

Sight

Below 30 weeks gestational age, a prem is not able to constrict her pupils to limit the amount of light coming into her eyes. This only works properly after about 34 weeks. Below 32 weeks, the eyelids also do not limit the entry of light. We need therefore to protect the prem's developing eyes from direct light exposure (9).

When she is on your chest with "tummy to mummy" with your shirt and blankets over you both, her eyes will be protected.

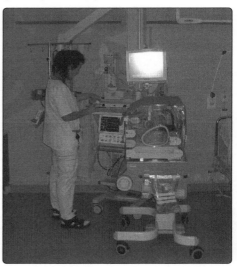

We also need to protect your prem's REM sleep (see the sleep cycling section). Your baby needs periods of darkness or low light in the NICU to help her regulate her own biological clock and get her day/night rhythm in place. Natural light is far better than artificial light, and fluorescent lights are bad for her as they flicker. Switch off lights not in use.

If she is in the incubator put dark covers on her eyes or place a dark cloth over the incubator.

It is important to keep a dim light in the NICU ward. If your baby needs phototherapy check that she has very dark, soft eye covers to protect her eyes, covering around the edges as well.

Individual personality or sensitivity

It is very important to remember that each baby is a wonderful individual with her own personality. Your own baby is unique, with her own likes and dislikes! She will react to things differently from another baby. This may be surprising to the nurses and doctors as it was not recognized before.

Watch your baby to see what she can do and support that; see what she cannot do, and help her. Look for her competence. Some babies can breathe on their own at 28 weeks gestational age, others can't. Some can co-ordinate sucking, swallowing and breastfeeding, while others at the same age need cup-feeding.

> **"Behaviour of the infant is its primary way to communicate" (Als)**

Watch your baby, especially her face, to pick up her own unique messages to you, which tell you how she is feeling. Read the small signs of your own baby being "disorganized"; signs that say "stop" or "give me a break or help me to calm down". If you are watching your baby in the incubator and can pick up the little signals of stress and respond to her quickly, you will help her to avoid becoming unstable or sick. Help her to self-regulate or find her balance by placing your hands on her and holding her still. You will know her better than anybody as you will spend hours watching her (10).

Premature babies are fragile and sensitive, and will show their stress in different ways. Different babies react differently to stimulation. Some are more sensitive and will quickly be overwhelmed. Mum, you will need to be sensitive to your baby's responses to you; be respectful and stop doing anything if she is becoming stressed (11).

> **If your prem is showing stress signals: stop and hold her still until her body calms down and she settles, her heart rate is normal and her body is still.**

"Clustering care", which means doing all procedures together with minimal handling, means that your baby can get longer rest times, and good sleep cycling. You can help her keep balanced by loving her and watching her carefully to see what she can cope with.

Some books will tell you to stimulate her with bright colours and voices, others will tell you not to over-stimulate her, and still other books will tell you to follow your instincts! This can be very confusing, and the truth lies in between. For example, if your baby was born at 32 weeks gestation, let her look at you, but don't talk at the same time. This may over-stimulate her.

A good general idea for prems is to do only ONE thing at a time at first. Give her small doses of stimulation and stop if she looks away or shows any of the stress signals. In time, she will cope with lots of messages at once. "Stop" – doing whatever has upset her – even talking to her or making eye contact can be too much for her. "Look" around – are there bright lights that may be hurting her eyes? "Listen" for loud noises that may have disturbed her.

> **Watch your baby!**

See the signs of a baby who is stressed and disorganized in the Separation & Stress chapter.

If your baby's oxygen level drops ("desaturation"), it can be bad for her brain. If this happens, do not handle her a lot. Calm containing and holding will help, however. Don't change nappies if she is upset and restless.

Don't watch the monitors – watch your little person. She needs you to learn to read her signals and to change what you do to make her feel better.

For example, if she gets unsettled or unstable when you are tube-feeding her, slow down the speed of flow of the milk.

If she is uncomfortable after a feed, maybe her tummy is too full (like you after a big dinner). Give her less milk at a time – remember her tiny stomach is only the size of a marble – and feed her more often.

Questions about your NICU

Light

▶ Does your NICU have bright lights or dim?...
▶ Are the lights dimmed at night to help your baby get a day/night rhythm?.................
▶ Do the nurses use dark cloths over the incubators?...

Noise

▶ Is the NICU full of loud noises?..
▶ Are loud noises, cell phones allowed?...
▶ Is there a noise monitor? ....
▶ Is there an awareness of speaking softly and are there reminder charts?...................

Here are some things to look for in your baby – find your own too.

What makes her cry?	
Does her body jerk when there is a loud sound?	
Does she turn towards your voice?	
Does she relax when you hold her close to you?	
Does she react to bright light?	
When do her eyes open most?	
Is she unsettled after she has eaten?	
Does she like to lie on her side?	
What makes your baby's oxygen level drop?(desaturation)	
What makes her scrunch up her face unhappily?	
Is she calmer if she is contained in a nest in the incubator?	
How does she react if you sing to her?	
What are her best times during the day?	
How long can she interact with you before getting too tired?	
What things that happen in the NICU does she react badly to?	
Does she react to strong smells?	
Does she sleep better on your chest or in the incubator?	
Is her breathing more regular when she is lying flat or up at an angle?	

Aim at these signs showing that your baby is peaceful.

- Her arms and legs are curled up in the flexed, fetal position.
- Her heart rate, breathing and oxygen saturation are even.
- Her skin colour is even.
- Her face looks relaxed.
- Her eyes open.
- Her hands are near her face.
- She may suck on her fist.
- Her hands are gently curled up and may be clasped together.
- She may hold on to your finger.

Contain arm + finger hold.

Maybe you could work with the nurses and put up a list of things that your baby is sensitive to on her incubator.

> **There are differences between prems born at different stages and these are important for your prem.**

These differences depend on how prematurely your baby was born (the gestational age). Remember that each baby is an individual, so she may be 32 weeks, but can be small for her age, or weaker. Here are three broad groups with some ideas for care.

Read whichever applies to your baby!

Near term (more than 36 weeks)

At nearly full term, babies are usually reasonably strong and able to cope without extra technology. The best care for them would be skin-to-skin contact. This SSC will help breastfeeding to start straight after birth, and the baby will be warm with a stable heart rate when she is on her mother. Avoiding separation is the best care.

Premature (32 – 36 weeks)

These babies are usually reasonably stable, and usually do well without lots of machinery. The prem is usually strong enough and developed enough to start breastfeeding straight after delivery. She can suck and swallow safely. Your prem will need mum's skin-to-skin contact to keep her temperature, heart rate and oxygen saturation stable. She will grow twice as fast in SSC compared to incubator care. Avoid separation by doing as much skin-to-skin contact as you can. This provides the best stability for her development and brain wiring.

   Skin-to-skin contact can still be done with all the monitors attached. The NICU nurses can help you to transfer the baby safely.

Very premature (<32w)

In SSC

If your baby is less than 32 weeks, her lungs are probably not developed enough to breathe yet and she may need technical support. You can still do skin-to-skin contact with all the machinery, but the staff of your NICU will need to be experienced to do this. Keep all the monitors attached during skin-to-skin contact, so that you and the staff will see how stable baby is. This will give an objective measure of how well she is coping.

In the incubator

Her brain still has a lot of developing to do, and you want to help your fragile tiny baby. Under 28 weeks of gestation the number of problems prems face is very much greater. Importantly, here you need to avoid her crying which increases blood pressure and places her at increased risk of a brain bleed. Also, do not lift her feet too high when you change her nappy.

   Do all you can with "developmental care" to help avoid stress for your prem. Being next to her and putting your hand on her back in the incubator may be all you can do for her at this stage, but she really needs you to be there with her. Talk gently to her.

   Importantly, the lights should be dimmed, as her pupils cannot constrict. Positioning and nesting are important (12).

> **Little things done early can make a huge difference later!**

Fine Print Page – Developmental care

All of these references are recommended reading, and practical to apply in neonatal care.

1. This and some of the articles that follow on this page, come from a hard cover journal, all of which deals with sensory environment, which is core to development and subsequent attachment.
2. NIDCAP was developed by Heidelise Als. A key concept is involvement of the family.
3. Another key concept is that the framework (synactive model) is holistic. The positive outcome does not come from doing one or two things, like covering incubators or nesting, but from the "total care package".
4. This is the largest study on NIDCAP to date, and provides a clear review of previous studies, and a good explanation of the principles of NIDCAP. It shows the improvement in long-term developmental care outcomes for prems given NIDCAP care.
5. Smell is far more important to the newborn than we realize!
6. The cloth idea might seem simplistic …and some may object to it being "unsterile"! Babies that get mum's milk have good immunity, and are calmed by her smell.
7. This article explains both the positive and harmful effects of sound in general,
8. Mother's voice is regulating: quote" The newborn shows heart rate decelerations in response to speech sounds. Early experience with voice has acute and enduring effects on the developing brain … with effects (on) development of the auditory system, as well as for later social and emotional development.."
9. Visual development is very complex … but one of the key aspects for the premature is ensuring sleep and protection from bright light, "Spontaneous synchronous retinal waves occur in preterm infants in the neonatal intensive care unit and must be protected, as they are critical for visual development."
10. This is a very hands-on and practical article by one of the very first NIDCAP pioneers.
11. This book describes the stress behaviours in detail.
12. Another practical paper, identifies 16 better care practices and discusses the practical implementation of each in detail, "containment and body flexion" is the first. http://www.nature.com/jp/journal/v27/n2s/pdf/7211843a.pdf

Reference List

(1) Browne JV. Early relationship environments: physiology of skin-to-skin contact for parents and their preterm infants. Clin Perinatol 2004 June;31(2):287-98, vii.
(2) Als H, Butler S. Newborn individualized developmental care and assessment program (NIDCAP) . Changing the furtue fior infants and families in intensive care nurseries. Early Childhood Services 2008;2(1):1-20.
(3) Als H. A synactive model of neonatal behavioral organization: framework for the assessment of neurobehavioral development in the premature infant and for support of infants and parents in the neonatal intensive care environment. Physical & Occupational Therapy in Pediatrics 1986;6(3/4):3-53.
(4) Peters KL, Rosychuk RJ, Hendson L, Cote JJ, McPherson C, Tyebkhan JM. Improvement of short-and long-term outcomes for very low birth weight infants: Edmonton NIDCAP trial. Pediatrics 2009;124:1009-20.
(5) Schaal B, Hummel T, Soussignan R. Olfaction in the fetal and premature infant: functional status and clinical implications. Clin Perinatol 2004 June;31(2):261-vii.
(6) Cernoch JM, Porter RH. Recognition of maternal axillary odors by infants. Child Dev 1985 December;56(6):1593-8.
(7) Gray L, Philbin MK. Effects of the neonatal intensive care unit on auditory attention and distraction. Clin Perinatol 2004 June;31(2):243-60.
(8) Fifer.W.P, Moon CM. The role of mother's voice in the organization of brain function in the newborn. Acta Paediatr 1994;Suppl 397:86-93.
(9) Graven SN. Early neurosensory visual development of the fetus and newborn. Clin Perinatol 2004 June;31(2):199-216, v.
(10) Lawhon G. Management of stress in premature infants. In: Angelini DJ, Whelan Knapp CM, Gibes RM, editors. Perinatal/Neonatal Nursing. A Clinical handbook. Boston: Blackwell Scientific Publications; 1986. p. 319-27.
(11) Madden SL. The preemie parents companion. Massachusetts: Harvard Common Press; 2000.
(12) Laudert S, Liu WF, Blackington S, Perkins B, Martin S, Millan-York E et al. Implementing potentially better practices to support the neurodevelopment of infants in the NICU. Journal of Perinatology 2007 December 2;27:S-5-S93.

TECHNOLOGY

Mum and Dad, it is normal to feel overwhelmed by all the machinery and monitors in the NICU, and you may feel helpless. She is your baby however, and you must have the right to be with her, to hold her on your naked chest (cover her back to keep her warm), to touch her and feed her.

DO NOT BE SCARED OFF BY THE MACHINES.

All of the machines may seem complicated and sophisticated, but the machines really do rather simple things and the basic concepts are NOT complicated.

Every baby is different but understanding the medical jargon may help you. The nurses and doctors often use abbreviations. You have a right to know this information. You are her parents, so find out as much about the technology as you can. Find out about her needs and set about providing them – this makes it easier to cope and begins to empower you to care for your baby.

For each section in this chapter, there are some simple explanations and "buzzwords" or technical jargon and abbreviations. There is also a table of basics and a space for your doctor to explain and fill in what your baby needed.

Resuscitation and birth period

Your baby has been born early and now no longer gets food, blood circulation and oxygen via the umbilical cord, so she has to get her own systems going. Some of these may not yet be fully developed. The hospital staff will need to assess what she will need help with in terms of machinery or technology.

At birth the staff will do an <u>APGAR score</u>, a 1–10 score of your baby's heart and lung condition. They will usually do this at 1, 5 and 10 minutes.

Your baby may need Cardio (heart) Pulmonary (lung) Resuscitation (CPR) to help to get the heart and lungs and breathing working.

Sometimes they need to intubate (put a tube into your baby's lungs) to help her breathe.

Sometimes babies are suctioned at birth. This is done less often these days, but it is done if there is fluid in the airways. The noise may sound worrying for parents.

<u>What resuscitation did your baby need?</u>

....

....

....

....

....

....

<u>Breathing and Oxygen</u>

Getting oxygen throughout the body needs three things:

▶ the heart to pump,

▶ the lungs to fill with air,

▶ and the haemoglobin in the blood to carry the oxygen to the body tissues.

Each of these can be supported.

The fetus inside the mother gets her oxygen from the mother via the placenta from the mother's bloodstream. When the baby is born the baby's lungs have to fill with air. The very first breath she takes does this fully. She doesn't need to cry to do this.

The lungs though may not be ready to inflate properly. Surfactant helps the lungs to inflate, but there is not enough in a prem. Steroids given to the mother two days before the birth will increase surfactant. The doctors may need to give artificial surfactant to the baby.

Baby under oxygen hood

Here is some of the technical help your premature baby may need for breathing:

Abbreviations:	Translated	Meaning
CPR	Cardio Pulmonary Resuscitation	This machine will help her breathe as her lungs have not developed enough to breathe
IPPV	Intermittent Positive Pressure Ventilation.	Helps the lungs which are elastic to inflate by blowing in air under pressure
	Oscillator.	Which is a high frequency ventilator
O_2 sats SaO_2	Oxygen Saturation	clip with a red light attached to her finger or toe for checking amount of oxygen in the blood. About 87–92% is good. (this also depends on the gestational age of the baby)
	Hood	A hood to cover the baby's head and give higher oxygen concentration
	Nasal Canula	Tiny pipe with holes going into the nostrils with extra oxygen
CPAP	Continuous Positive Airways Pressure	Extra push of pressure to get oxygen to the blood
	Surfactant	Acts like a type of foam to help the lungs to inflate properly. It keeps the lungs soft and elastic so they can easily open and close

Heart and circulation

For a prem, the heart is usually competent.

The heart has already been pumping in the womb, but now some valves direct the blood in the big blood vessels of the heart to flow in a different direction. Inside you your baby would be getting oxygen dissolved in her blood through the placenta and the umbilical cord. Suddenly, her body has to try to get her own oxygen and her heart has to circulate it around her body.

Your baby may be linked to a heart monitor. Many parents of prems spend those first agonizingly long weeks in the NICU gazing at the monitors ready to react if the red light flashes.

Heart Rate (HR) – this is how fast the heart is beating to pump blood around the body. The heart rate needs to be fast enough to circulate oxygen and food. The heart rate of a tiny prem will be faster than an adult's and it may also be very irregular. Initially the range is 120–160. An irregular heart rate may be evidence of instability. Small changes in heart rate are normal. The heart rate is usually easy to measure.

Blood Pressure (BP) – this needs to be high enough to push the blood to the tissues, but not so high that it bursts the blood vessels. Blood pressure is more difficult to measure than the heart rate. Medicines can be used to increase or decrease the heart rate, and increase blood pressure, or to help the heart muscle itself.

HR	Heart rate	
	Bradycardia	Slow heart rate
	Tachycardia	Fast heart rate
BP	Blood pressure	
	hypotension	Low blood pressure
	hypertension	High blood pressure
Your Baby		

Fluid management

To carry the oxygen we need blood which means fluids.

The fetus gets all her fluid from the placenta.

The newborn baby must drink.

The premature newborn cannot drink enough! (The premature baby CAN safely swallow as she has been swallowing amniotic fluids since 16 weeks gestation.)

When a full-term baby is born, she has 10% extra weight which is liquid. This liquid is to help the baby cope for the first three days until her mother's breast milk has started to come through properly. Newborns often lose weight for the first three days as they lose that extra fluid.

A baby may need all these drips

For the premature this early weight loss needs to be managed carefully as breastfeeding takes longer to get started.

Premature babies are often unable to keep their fluid balance right. They lose a lot of fluid easily and dehydrate through the skin, so their body may need to be covered by a sheet of thin plastic to hold in the water. The air inside the incubator is humidified to prevent evaporation loss. Skin-to-skin contact also prevents water loss through the skin. (You may be worried to find that your baby has a splint on the arm that has a drip. This is to stabilise the

Baby's body covered in plastic.

drip line, and does not mean that her arm is broken!)

The kidneys "clean" all the fluid in the body but they are only mature at 3 months after a full term birth.

Your baby may need a drip for fluids. This can be placed in several ways (see "Lines" in the chart below). Various fluids can be given through these lines.

	Breastmilk	This is the best medicine any premature baby can be given!
	Neonatal maintenance solution	A carefully balanced liquid for prems.
TPN	Total Parenteral Nutrition	The tiny baby is fed into the veins, ie not through the stomach.
	a peripheral line	A drip directly into the veins of the hand, arm or foot or scalp.
	a central line	a tiny tube into a bigger vein, this lasts longer.
	an umbilical line	A drip put into the baby's umbilicus, this can be used for the first few days.
	arterial line	Sicker babies need to get fluid directly into the arteries
	enteral line	This tube goes straight into the stomach eg a naso-gastric tube - this is a good way to provide fluids.
Your own baby's treatment		

Food management

> **Your prem's gut is very immature. Actually, the gut is biologically immature until 6 months of age. Your baby's gut depends on human milk; from 28 weeks gestational age mother's milk is good. Any foreign substance causes harm to the immature gut.**

In the womb, your baby would be getting exactly the right food from mum; it is dissolved in the blood in the placenta and carried to her in the umbilical cord. Inside mum, her stomach was working, but did not have much going through it. When your baby is born, she must eat and swallow for herself. Though her swallowing muscles are ready, the rest of her body may not be ready.

So she may need either a **naso-gastric tube** (NGT) into her nose or an **oro-gastric tube** (OGT) through her mouth straight into the stomach. The tube will be is fixed to her face with tape and she will be given her food through it. **Either NGT or OGT is called gavage feeding**. Your expressed breast milk is what she needs most to help her immunity to develop and to provide the food that her brain needs the most.

Your baby needs a supply of brain fuel: this is critical. She also needs body fuel for her metabolism and she needs extra calories for growth. Your baby will have a growth chart in

This baby has a 'stoma'

the NICU. In the first few days, her weight will probably go down a little. After this, you hope to see it going up. There may be dips now and then, but do not panic or be discouraged. Simple things may change: for example, was your daughter weighed before or after a meal, before or after urinating, before a nappy change, or at a different time of day. There are many variables. Try to see the big trend.

Abbreviations:	Translated	Meaning
EBM	Expressed Breast milk:	the mother is encouraged to express or squeeze out or pump her breast milk to be fed to her own baby.
MOM	Mothers own milk:	the best!
HMB	Human Milk Bank:	If a mother cannot supply milk, babies sometimes get pasteurised milk from other mothers.
AIF	Artificial Infant Formula:	dried cows' milk, with additives.
LC	Lactation Consultant:	someone specially trained to help with breast feeding.
	FM 85 calcium supplement:	this is given if baby does not grow for more than 3 days.
NGT	naso-gastric tube:	your baby will be given her liquid food or breast milk through a tube going through her nose straight to her stomach.

OGT	oro-gastric tube:	your baby will be given her liquid food through a tube going through her mouth straight to her stomach.
	hypoglycaemia:	low blood sugar level..
	hyperglycaemia	high blood sugar level.
Your Baby		

Temperature management

Warmth – in the mother's womb, the baby's body temperature is kept constant.

When the full term baby is born she needs to regulate her own temperature and can usually manage this. Above 2200 g, temperature control starts to work better. If the baby weighs less than 1800 g, the body mass is too small for the surface area and she cannot maintain her own temperature.

Even if the baby is bigger, a cold environment or draft or evaporation can lower her temperature dangerously. This is why babies should not be bathed in the first hour of life – this hot water and cold air destabilises their temperature. If the baby gets cold, the surfactant in the lungs stops working.

If the baby is separated from her mother, her temperature will fluctuate chaotically. The control centre in her brain will reduce her core temperature so that she uses up less of her essential fat supplies or calories to keep her temperature constant. It takes food energy to keep the temperature normal, so these calories are then not available for growth.

There are two technical words linked to temperature. **Hypothermia** means the body is too cold; **hyperthermia** means the body is too hot. A healthy temperature range is 36 to 37,2° C.

Incubators are used to keep prems warm. This is done in a variety of ways: with closed incubators, overhead heaters, infrared lights, open incubators and water beds.

> **The mother's chest regulates the baby's temperature better than any incubator ever could do. Skin-to-skin contact keeps the temperature in the higher range and constant.**

Mum, if you put your naked baby skin-to-skin on your chest, your body can naturally warm by 2°C to warm your cold baby and your temperature can drop by 1°C to cool her if she is warm. This is called "Thermal Synchrony".

Research has shown that the mother's breasts act independently! If there are twins who have different temperatures, one breast cools, while the other warms. Aren't mothers' bodies amazing!

Your own baby			

Monitoring and protection of the premature baby

Your baby has been born too early and is very fragile. The NICU staff will monitor your baby to make sure that there is progress, and to make sure that your baby is well and protected.

You may find your eyes fixed to the monitors, but remember that your own sense of your baby's well-being is the best monitor there is. You are her constant carers, while the nurses change in shifts and doctors come and go. She is your child and you will be the most sensitive to small changes in her condition. Look at her colour; listen to her breathing, movements, awake-ness, eye contact, restlessness and skin texture. Tell the nurse if you notice even a small change. You, Mum and Dad, can be the most sensitive monitors of your baby's progress.

> **Your own gut feeling of your baby's present condition is very likely to be correct!**

Keep asking about the charts, and realize that there will be ups and downs. Also try to learn how to check if the monitors are properly attached. The graphs on the monitors will go up and down and show irregularities; this may be difficult for you emotionally. Try to look for the bigger trends, rather than the small ups and downs.

Laboratory and other tests

Some of the basic tests are X-rays (XR) and ultrasounds (US). These look at the bones and basic organs of the baby. Blood tests check blood sugar levels, electrolytes and other chemicals in the blood. Bilirubin is one of the most commonly done tests. Bilirubin increases if the liver can not remove the contents of broken down blood cells fast enough. If the bilirubin level is too high, it can damage the brain. If her bilirubin is raised, your baby will need to be under phototherapy lights, which help break down the bilirubin.

Some tests on newborns are "<u>non-invasive</u>" like an ECG. These tests can be done when we need essential information and there is no risk for the child.

Other tests are "<u>minimally invasive</u>". Here the doctors and nurses have to balance the risk of not having information

Baby in phototherapy on mother

with the risk of harm while getting the information. For example, a heel prick to collect blood may be needed. The baby can cope with one or two times, but by the time they leave the NICU, some babies have had 750 heel pricks and it is very likely that this causes harm.

Other tests are "<u>invasive</u>". We know that the risk for harm is high, but they may be needed for survival, e.g. an arterial catheter.

As her parents, you should be consulted about all the tests your baby needs and be given time to ask questions about them, especially if you know the risk of harm is high. You need to give your consent – a signed consent form is needed in some hospitals.

Any painful procedure should have pain relief. Remember that skin-to-skin contact and breastfeeding both relieve pain so use them together when painful procedures are done for your baby.

Monitoring includes checking the various chemicals in your baby's blood. Some of these tests can be done with a small amount of blood from a heel prick; others will need more blood drawn from a vein, and blood gases are usually measured from an artery.

These are some of the tests that can be done on your baby in the NICU. The tests and their names vary between hospitals and countries. You could fill in your baby's tests below.

	Weight	usually done daily.
	Head circumference	weekly.
	Length	measured weekly in some hospitals, others do not see it as important at all.
Dx	Dextrose checks	these are done hourly for the first three hours, then 3 hourly for 24 hours to check blood sugar levels.
	Electrolytes	usually done only if baby is on CPAP or ventilator.
	Blood gases	these check oxygen and carbon dioxide in the blood. These are usually done only if baby is on CPAP or a ventilator.

		Haematocrit	tests iron; done at birth, then weekly.
BR		Bilirubin test	done if the baby is becoming jaundiced; it is more commonly done on O positive and Rhesus negative blood group babies. The test is done 6 hours after delivery and repeated after 12 hours.
CRP		C Reactive Protein	important if there is an infection.
LFT		Liver function test	done weekly if the staff are concerned about infection or if liver is enlarged.
CaPO4 Mg		Calcium phosphate	may be done if the baby does not grow in the first week and the staff suspect rickets.
FBC		Full blood count	done only if infection is suspected.
		Urine test	protein checked if infection is suspected.
		Ultrasound of head	done every third day if the head circumference increases and the staff suspect IVH (intraventricular haemorrhage).
CXR		Chest X Rays	
AXR		Abdominal X rays	
US		Ultrasound	also used in "echo" as in echocardiography, Doppler, etc ...
ECG		Electrocardiogram	measures the electrical activity in the heart.
Your Baby			

Monitoring usually includes protecting the physical needs of the body, but often has not considered protecting the brain from stress. The baby also needs immunity which includes the antibodies in her blood and breast milk which also provides her food. On top of all these is emotional security which is vital for all newborns and even more so for a fragile premature baby.

Most importantly, she needs the immune protection provided by her mother's milk. About 90% of the contents of human breast milk are for protection.

Inside the mother the fetus is protected by the muscles of the uterus. Sounds are muted, it is dark and warm, and sensations are mostly calm and pleasurable. The baby is in a secure, fixed place, in close relationship to her mother.

Mother <u>IS</u> baby's protection

More and more modern research is showing how the mother provides all the aspects of protection and that a baby needs continuity with her mother for healthy development.

> **If a baby is separated from her mother when she is born, she feels completely unprotected, vulnerable, alone, insecure and stressed.**
> **Technology may be needed to assist your baby to cope with the changes at birth, as an add-on, but not as a substitute for Mum.**
> **The premature baby is even more dependent on her mother.**

The technology that has developed in the NICU separates a premature baby from her mother. The lights are too bright for her eyes, she has no way of closing her ears to all the many voices and beeping machine sounds in a busy NICU.

She needs protection against the pain of heel pricks, protection against over-stimulation and immunity against bacterial, viral and yeast infections. She needs protection against stress and the emotional trauma of separation for correct brain development. Her sensory needs are for "soft care" (see the section on developmental care).

Here is space to fill in any extra abbreviations below that are used in your NICU.
Ask the staff to fill them in and explain to you.

> **There has not been a randomised controlled trial done on the safety of the incubator. You, Mum and Dad, are a far superior quality incubator in every way.**

Again: DO NOT BE INTIMIDATED by the machinery.

Here are some practical things that you can do for your tiny baby as you sit with her for hours in the NICU, staring at the monitors or at her in an incubator.

▷ If an alarm goes off on your baby's machinery, it is for a reason. Do not ignore the alarm. You may need to go and call a nurse to ask why the alarm has gone off.

▷ Check the temperature controls of the incubator. If the temperature is above 37,5°C, you should alert a nurse.

▷ If your baby is having phototherapy for jaundice, always check that her eyes are properly covered with thick or dark cloth.

▷ The clip of the oxygen saturation probe with the red light needs to be moved every hour, moving from left to right hand to right foot to left foot.

▷ If your baby is on a drip or "intravenous line", check that the nurse has always recorded the date and time when the drip was started.

▷ Check that the drip site is not swollen and the skin around it is not red. Check that the fingers are not swelling. Sometimes there are small bubbles in the drip line, but there should not be big bubbles.

Often NICU babies need lots of machinery

Now here is a reality check!

Each hospital or NICU has different policies and routines and treatments and a professional team is there to help you and your baby to survive. Survival is the most urgent, important aspect for the NICU team – but increasingly we are aware that the quality of survival is important. This is your important work, mum and dad!

Mum and Dad make the difference to the quality of survival. This is measured in neurodevelopment.

Appreciate the NICU team but realize that they cannot replace you as your baby's parent. You can and should politely insist on being there as much as possible and touching her. If a hospital wants to exclude you from NICU or not let you touch your baby, consider changing to a more humane hospital!

The team can help your prem to survive physically, but to make the best of her fragile neurological situation, she is primed to need you.

To encourage you, answer the following questions (put this into words or give a percentage).

1. How much of this did you know before your baby was born? ....

2. How much of this did you know after one week? ....

3. How much of this did you know when you were discharged from the hospital?.................

....

You have already learnt a huge amount which will help you to cope so that you can help your baby in the best way possible!

Does your hospital or NICU
▶   allow you to be part of the caring team? ....
▶   allow you to be central to the caring team?..
▶   answer your questions?...
▶   explain what treatment they are giving and why?..

Please let us know how we can improve this information to help other parents.

email to jill@kangaroomothercare.com
or write to: Jill Bergman, 8 Francis Road, Pinelands, 7405, Cape Town, South Africa

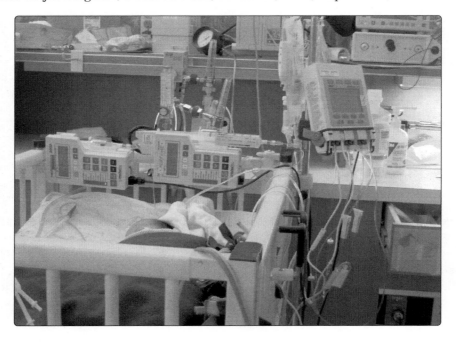

PROBLEMS PREMS MAY FACE IN THE NICU

Coming in to the NICU and seeing all of the machines and tubes around tiny babies will probably feel really scary for you as parents. It will all be new and unfamiliar.

Try to ask questions of the staff and find out as much as you can about problems that your own baby may have. You will find many different people in the NICU. Some nurses don't want to give you too many details of what could go wrong. Other staff members feel that it is best to tell parents everything so that they can cope and face the worst. Ask the nurses to explain what is happening. Generally the more you know, the better you cope as parents of a prem and can help care for your baby. The more you understand, the more you can help. Try to trust. This is not to worry you, but to inform you.

Firstly, do NOT presume that any or all of these apply to your baby!

There are many technical terms for the common problems of prematurity; this is a very simplified alphabetical list of the most common problems for everyday people to understand. Because the terms are so long, nurses and doctors often use abbreviations.

After the list you will see some of the longer-term problems prems <u>may</u> face as they grow.

This list is not for reading, it is for looking up something and is in <u>alphabetical order</u>. It is also for you to ask your doctor or nurse for details that apply to *your* baby and write these in the spaces at the end.

	Air leaks	Air gets into the chest cavity around the lungs. This is a pneumothorax and can be an emergency.
	Apnoea	Pauses in breathing lasting more than 20 seconds. The baby "forgets" to breathe as her brain is immature. The heart rate slows and the baby becomes more "blue". She may need caffeine or theophylline to stimulate her and she often needs an apnoea monitor She may need CPAP or medicine to help her breathe. This can be very scary for parents.
A's and B's	Apnoea and Bradycardia	Apnoea: lack of breathing (sometimes stimulated with caffeine). Bradycardia: very slow heart rate.
	Anaemia	The baby may have too few red blood cells which carry oxygen to the body. She may need a blood transfusion.
	Asystole	The heart stops beating.
BPD	Bronchopulmonary dysplasia	The lungs of of a prem are immature so the baby needs extra oxygen. Diuretics may be used to help get fluid off the lungs; bronchodilators may be used to open the airways or a ventilator may be needed.

	Cardiac arrest	The heart stops beating.
CP	Cerebral Palsy	There is damage to the brain before or during birth. There can be weakness of arms, legs or face, but this is often not seen until later in life.
	Collapsed lung	This is caused by a hole in a lung. It may need an "underwater drain" into the chest cage which bubbles under water to open the lung.
GER	Gastro- oesophageal reflux	This is vomiting up food (called "spitting up" in the USA). Reflux can also be acidic food in the oesophagus that causes pain.
	Hydrocephalus	This is "water in the head". It is actually spinal fluid in the ventricles of the brain. The baby's head may grow too fast and there is increased pressure on the brain. The baby may need a shunt to get rid of the extra fluid.
	Hyperbilirubinemia	See jaundice
	Hyperglycaemia	This is difficulty with sugar balance: prem babies often have blood sugar levels that are too high.
	Hypoglycaemia	Prems can have blood sugar levels that are too low.
IVH	Intraventricular haemorrhage	This is a brain bleed because the blood vessels in the brain are tiny and fragile. The blood seeps into spaces in the brain. Often ultrasounds are done to check this. Complications are more likely with grade 3 and 4 IVH. The baby will need careful checking over time to monitor her development.
	Jaundice or hyperbilirubinemia	The baby's skin sometimes seems yellow because old red blood cells are broken down in the liver and the body cannot get rid of bilirubin, the waste product. She may need phototherapy under ultraviolet lights. About 50% of prems need ultraviolet light; only about 20% of full term babies need phototherapy.
NEC	Necrotising enterocolitis	Prem babies have immature stomachs and sometimes an infection can cause part of the intestines to die. The baby will be given antibiotics and may be fed through a vein and watched carefully. Giving the colostrum, the first breast milk, prevents this problem.
PDA	Patent ductus arteriosus	Before birth, the baby does not need to breathe air through the lungs. The PDA lets blood flow directly to the fetus' body instead of to the lungs. The blood vessel joining the aorta to the pulmonary artery has a duct or valve which closes at birth; in a prem this may not have closed yet.
	Pneumonia	Lung infection

		Pneumothorax	This is caused by a hole in a lung. it may need an "underwater drain" into the chest cage which bubbles under water to open the lung.
PPHN		Persistent pulmonary hypertension	Blood vessels around the lungs are small and tight. They should be relaxed and open so the baby can get enough oxygen.
PVL		Periventricular leukomalacia	This refers to damage to brain tissue caused by decreased blood flow.
RDS		Respiratory distress syndrome	A prem baby's lungs are immature and cannot produce surfactant, The baby may breathe too fast or "grunt". She may need extra oxygen by CPAP or breathing machine, a ventilator or respirator.
ROP		Retinopathy of prematurity	Prems' eyes are very vulnerable and blood vessels can grow abnormally in the retina. Keep the lights dimmed. She may need eye checks at 4-6 weeks and may need glasses later.
		Seizures	A prem's nervous system is immature and there may be muscle spasm or twitching. This can be caused by low blood sugar, mineral imbalance, infections or brain bleeds.
		Sepsis	The body responds to bacterial or viral infection with inflammation. Antibiotics and intensive care are needed.
SIDS		Sudden Infant Death Syndrome	This can affect any child, but as prems' lungs are so fragile, they are more likely to have SIDS. Breastfeeding, lying the baby on her back, safe sleeping and NO SMOKING for parents of prems can help prevent SIDS.
TTN		Transient Tachypnea of the newborn	The baby breathes too fast because of pneumonia or infection and she needs to be given more oxygen.
Your Baby			

LONG TERM PROBLEMS PREMS MAY FACE & HOW SKIN-TO-SKIN CONTACT CAN HELP

Modern medical science has advanced so much that far more very tiny babies of 26 or even 22 weeks gestation are surviving. There are still questions as to the QUALITY of that survival and how many problems this tiny baby and her parents will have to cope with as she grows (1).

Prems have not had an ideal start as they were born too early. It is known that babies born premature have in the past had far less developed brains than full term babies. **Now we know that this need not be so.** Even extremely premature babies can do very well.

If a baby is born before 26 weeks there is a high risk of major developmental problems which may cause difficulties or delays later on. Under 24 or 25 weeks of gestation the number of problems prems face is very much greater (2).

> **"I would hope that people understand that being born early is a very, very serious business, that survival is not high, and that should children survive, their likelihood of having life-long problems – particularly in respect of learning – is high".**
>
> **"We need to do all that we can to find ways to bridge the baby's developmental gap and to nurture healthy brain development outside the womb."**
>
> *Professor Kate Costeloe* **(3)**

Holding your baby in skin-to-skin contact can help bridge this gap.

You as a parent will want to do all you can to minimize these problems. In the past prem babies have had a one in ten risk of cerebral palsy, a quarter may need help at school and have lower IQ. 40% of survivors have moderate to severe problems in brain development. Interestingly, boys are twice as likely to have problems later than girls (2).

This list is not to scare or depress you and <u>none</u> may apply to your baby, but if your expectations are realistic it is sometimes easier to cope. Facing the issues and having information about them may help you to cope better. Even more importantly, it will help show you how important it is that you are with your tiny baby holding her skin-to-skin to help her development to prevent problems later on. This is where this workbook began: "If only I had known, I would have done things differently..."

A common question is, "What can I expect in terms of development?"

Let's look at mental, physical and emotional development for separated babies compared to those in skin-to-skin contact.

Mental Development

Separated prems are at greater risk of

- ▶ brain bleeds (IVH) from stress and separation from their mothers;
- ▶ less brain development (1;4) and
- ▶ fewer neural pathways.

They are also at greater risk of developing learning and attention problems like ADD, ADHD (5;6) and possibly autism spectrum disorder (ASD).

Skin-to-skin care can help protect your baby. In the first days after birth, your baby held in skin-to-skin contact is calm and unstressed, and her brain is being wired for health. Also she does not cry, and therefore is less likely to have a brain bleed.

Developmentally, skin-to-skin contact is important over the first months for the "approach" brain pathways. Being with your baby will protect her sleep for healthy brain wiring; protect her eyes from bright lights; her ears from loud sounds; her nose from strong smells and her skin from rough handling and pain. All of these will protect her brain from the bad effects of stress.

Physical Development

Separated prems are at greater risk of

- cerebral palsy,
- delayed motor development,
- delayed speech development,
- feeding problems,
- blindness, or
- deafness (1).

If a prem lies on her back in an incubator for a month or two with her legs flopped out sideways, her hips may be rotated outwards, which could make crawling, and later walking, more difficult. Often a prem will walk with her toes turned outward. This could cause her to be teased, which further lowers her self-esteem in later years. Her motor skills of smiling, sitting, crawling, walking, speaking may well be delayed because of low muscle tone.

If she lies on her back in an incubator, her chest muscles can stretch and her back muscles shrink, and she may not even be able to get her arms to midline. This can make it harder for her to push herself up from her tummy and learn to crawl later. Delaying crawling can delay her speech development and mathematics ability. Often nothing is done until the child reaches preschool age. Start supporting her development in the NICU and you will have far fewer problems later.

Lying on her back can make her head flatter.

Skin-to-skin care can help protect your baby in the first days after birth. She will not be as stressed so her heart rate, blood pressure and breathing and temperature will stay more constant. She will start breastfeeding earlier, absorb her food better and so grow faster. Holding her upright and flexed on your chest helps the spine to learn to balance and increases muscle tone. If she is in an incubator, positioning her comfortably can make a huge difference.

Skin-to-skin contact and breastfeeding go together so here is a small note about the long-term benefits of breastfeeding. The action of suckling from the breast is needed to strengthen her jaw muscles and shape her jaw and mouth for later speech development and straight teeth The American Academy of Paediatrics recommends that mothers exclusively breastfeed their infants up to six months of age (7), and that nursing for a year or more will give a baby the "full benefits of breastfeeding," which include cutting rates of illnesses such as ear infections and diarrhoea and reducing the risk of childhood obesity. Babies should be breastfed for 2 years to grow to their maximum brain growth.

Emotional Development

Separated prems have spent a lot of time alone in an incubator in NICU, and so are stressed and dissociate emotionally. They may not bond or make good attachment to their parents or to others very easily. This can cause them huge problems emotionally and socially throughout their lives.

Skin-to-skin care can help your baby as she will feel emotionally safe, calm and loved. You provide your baby with the only familiar constant to give her emotional security, and help her catch up on what she has missed On your chest your prem can reach stability more easily (self-regulate). By putting her in the fetal position with her arms close to her chest and near her mouth you will help your prem to self-comfort and stabilize her body and her emotions. Your voice talking and singing to her will be reassuring.

Mum and Dad, your baby will trust you and feel safe with you and bond with you, and so be secure enough to bond with an increasing number of people, starting with family and friends. This will help her to build healthy relationships and will have long term benefits throughout her life.

Skin-to-skin contact between a baby and adoptive parents can have a hugely positive impact on bonding and building trust.

These simple things can have a profound impact on minimizing problems later on. If this means taking time off work for a few weeks to be in the NICU with your baby, do it. It can save you many months or years of problems later. It is a very worthwhile investment of time! If parents have to work, having one constant care-giver can provide a good base for development.

Some studies have even suggested that working parents can give a child the basic bonding time that she needs for healthy development by allowing her to co-sleep with them.

> There are many things that your prem can catch up over the first few years. Early professional help can make a huge difference to your baby's outcome. Get a physiotherapist involved AS EARLY AS POSSIBLE. He or she can draw up a set of exercises and activities for you to work on with your baby as early as you can. This can start with infant massage, and go on to tiny exercises in the NICU. The first few weeks and months of a baby's life are crucial.

Get help early

Remember that the baby has the most brain cells or neurons at 28 weeks gestation. These neurons are branching and connecting at synapses and are busiest in the first year of life. The "metabolic activity" in the brain is highest until 3 years of life; after this it slows down. Focus on supporting your baby in these first three years. **Do not wait** to discover problems at preschool, it will be very much more difficult then.

Some say that prems are behind and will "catch up" to their normal developmental milestones by two or three years. Others say that prems never fully catch up. The truth is somewhere in between, and will often depend on the individual baby. Expect delays!

It may feel like there is a long road ahead of you: ask for help from family and friends and health professionals; get advice; join with other parents of prems, read about prematurity; BE there for your baby. She needs your love; she needs you to be her champion. Work together and keep talking as a couple or family. Your prem needs as much help as she can get to make up for her early start. Most of all, she needs YOU, her parents, close to her, and your love can help to pull her through this rough start to life.

Ask for help from family and friends.

Fine Print Page – Long term problems prems may face

1. This articles reviews cerebral palsy primarily, and then more broadly developmental outcomes from very low birth weight babies. "VLBW infants remain at substantial risk for a wide spectrum of long-term morbidity including cerebral palsy (CP), mental retardation, developmental delay, school problems, behavioural issues, growth failure, and overall poor health status."
2. The smaller the babies, (<1000g) the worse the long term outcomes, but not always!
3. The EPICURE study from the UK is one of the most rigorous, with long term follow-up data.
4. An MRI study of brains of preterm infants, showing that they have not grown as they would have in the uterus.
5. ADD and ADHD approximately 3 times more common in prems.
6. Cognitive impairment is also related to decreasing gestational age at birth.
7. Breastfeeding and breast milk are protective.

Reference List

(1) Wilson-Costello D. Is there evidence that long-term outcomes have improved with intensive care? Seminars In Fetal & Neonatal Medicine 2007 October 16;12(5):344-54.

(2) Vohr BR, Wright LL, Dusick AM, Mele L, Verter J, Steichen JJ et al. Neurodevelopmental and functional outcomes of extremely low birth weight infants in the National Institute of Child Health and Human Development Neonatal Research Network, 1993-1994. Pediatrics 2000 June;105(6):1216-26.

(3) Costeloe K, Wood NS Gibson AT, Hennessy EM, Marlow N, Wilkinson AR. The EPICure study: associations and antecedents of neurological and developmental disability at 30 months of age following extremely preterm birth. Archives of Disease in Childhood -- Fetal & Neonatal Edition 2005 March;90(2):F134-F140.

(4) Inder TE, Warfield SK, Wang H, Huppi PS, Volpe JJ. Abnormal cerebral structure is present at term in premature infants. Pediatr 2005;115(2):286-94.

(5) Botting N, Powls A, Cooke RWI. Attention deficit hyperactivity disorders and other psychiatric outcomes in very low birth weight children at 12 years. J Child Psychol Psychiatry 1997;38(8):931-41.

(6) Cooke RW, Foulder-Hughes L. Growth impairment in the very preterm and cognitive and motor performance at 7 years. Arch Dis Child 2003;88(6):482-7.

(7) American Academy of Pediatric : Section on Breastfeeding. Breastfeeding and the use of human milk. American Academy of Pediatrics 2005;115(2):496-506.

HOW FRIENDS AND FAMILY CAN HELP

The birth of a child is a wonderful thing to happen in any family. The birth of a prem can be very difficult and brings its own mixture of joy, sadness and worry.

Parents, do ask for help!!

Grandparents can be a huge support.

Ask your family and friends to support you in whatever ways they can. They can help by not coming in to the NICU as this will be stressful for your baby and other babies there and bring in unnecessary germs.

Friends and family can have a huge role to play in coming alongside the parents of a premature infant.

It is often very difficult to repeat all the news of your baby. Give details of your prem's progress to one family member or friend. Everyone else can contact them and not disturb you. You can be cushioned in this way. Maybe you could get that person to send out a weekly email with a photo.

Parents do not try to be strong and cope on your own.

There are people who want to and can help you.

There is little that friends and family can do to help the prem baby directly, but here are some practical ideas from parents of prems themselves of what they would like help with!

Some things to do

▶ Offer practical support, e.g. being with the older siblings of the prem while Mum and Dad to go to the hospital.
▶ Grannies, aunts and friends can be a huge help by being stand-in caregivers for older siblings at home.
▶ Let the parents talk freely.
▶ Offer to do washing.
▶ Offer to take the siblings to school.
▶ Give support.
▶ Phone and ask how you can help or send a text message on a mobile phone. Parents can read this when it suits them. Don't expect an answer!
▶ Email your support.
▶ Offer to hold the baby while Mum sleeps. She will often feel too tired to "entertain you".
▶ Cook meals and answer phones, especially when the prem baby gets home.
▶ Offer to go shopping.
▶ Later, baby-sit when the prem is bigger – encourage Mum and Dad to go out for coffee together.

Some things to avoid

▶ Do not all go and visit the NICU – that takes too many foreign germs into the hospital and will stress the tiny baby.
▶ Don't ask if the baby will survive – the parents and doctors do not know and it is a huge worry for them.
▶ Don't ask lots of questions.
▶ Don't give lots of "advice".
▶ Do not take photographs with a flash as it will hurt the prem's eyes.
▶ Do not ask how long she will be in NICU – the parents and nurses do not know.
▶ Do not blame the parents as if it was their "fault" that they had a prem.
▶ Don't tell parents to "be strong" or "forget your baby for now and come out with us".
▶ Do not pretend that the baby does not exist, especially if she died. The prem was a very real person for that mother and father and always will be. Do not say, "you can always have another baby."
▶ Don't visit the parents when you are sick.
▶ Do not visit in the first weeks after the prem gets home. Let the family settle down at home first. Be sensitive to their needs.
▶ Do not be offended if the parents will not let you hold their prem baby. They have fought for her life and she feels more secure with them.
▶ Do not <u>ever</u> smoke in the same room as a prem. It can increase her risk of SIDS and she will be much more likely to get infections.
▶ Do not take offence if parents of prems seem irritable or angry with you. They are coping with an extremely stressful situation and need your support.

GOING HOME

When can my baby go home or be "discharged"?

This is very individual and depends on how early your prem was born, if she needed oxygen or surgery. Different hospitals have different measures or criteria for when a prem is ready to go home, for example when she is a certain weight or gestational age.

You can go home when

▶ you, the parents feel confident to care for your prem baby alone;

▶ your baby is exclusively breastfeeding, or she is feeding properly from breast or a cup;

▶ she is gaining weight continuously;

▶ she can keep her own body temperature normal;

▶ her heart and lungs are working properly;

▶ home is safe and mother has support and follow-up care.

Ideally, parents should have already been doing all the care for some time.

Many hospitals have a "rooming in" time for 24 hours for parents to learn all the care of their prem. Do ask for this so that you can care for all of the needs of your prem while you still have the support of the NICU staff, so that you can gain confidence.

Important

Your tiny baby is still premature and should not be left alone at home. She will still need very "intensive care" but from you, not from machines. Carrying your baby skin-to-skin in a KangaCarrier or sling will help you to continue to give your baby the best care while doing your home chores.

Going home may bring up a mixture of feelings in you. It is an exciting but sometimes scary time. You might feel <u>relieved</u> that you're home and not having to go to the hospital every day. Sometimes your prem has been in the NICU for many weeks, so it is a huge adjustment for you as parents to be completely responsible for her full time care, 24 hours a day. You may feel tired as there are no nurses to be care-givers while you take a break. Your prem baby may need to feed 10–14 times a day!

You may feel anxious that there are no nurses to support you or even monitors, and you may be worried that you may not be able to cope.

You may find yourself always worrying about your baby and often checking that she is breathing properly. You can sometimes feel lonely or isolated now that you are alone at home after the busy NICU. All of these are normal reactions! Be kind to yourself!

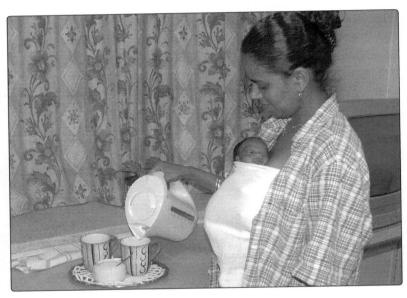

Going home checklists

Do you know how to

- give your baby all the care she needs;
- feed her as often as possible;
- change her nappy or diaper;
- calm your baby;
- give her a bath;
- give her medicines;
- put her safely in car seat (prems are too small for normal car seats – roll towels at the sides);
- do baby CPR;
- use the equipment;
- work the apnoea monitor if she needs oxygen?

Do you know

▶ if all your baby's immunizations and tests have been done;

▶ who her doctor will be;

▶ what immunizations she needs;

▶ know if / when tests need to be done, e.g., eye, hearing, ultrasound?

Have you got

▶ support at home

▶ safety numbers – Doctor, NICU, Lactation Consultants, social workers, clinics,

▶ all the prem clothes that you need (they need to be SOFT inside for her delicate skin);

▶ prem diapers/nappies (as small as possible);

▶ a breast pump if you need it;

▶ a discharge summary from the hospital of your baby's treatments, etc;

▶ a list of follow-up appointments at the clinic and for the 18 week corrected age check up;

▶ all her medicines if she needs any?

Some ideas for when you get home

▶ Rest at home.

▶ Make time to bond with your baby.

▶ Try to make home peaceful.

▶ Make your prem's "playtime" with siblings short – she needs to rest and sleep to grow.

▶ Keep the home temperature constant.

▶ If your prem is sweating, take off her clothes.

▶ You and the family should wash your hands often. Visitors especially need to wash their hands.

▶ Get a phone answering machine.

▶ No "pass the parcel" with visitors – keep your prem skin-to-skin on your chest.

Your ideas (your discharge nurse can help you here):

....

....

....

....

....

....

....

> ## The best advice I got when I had a newborn baby was:
>
> ## SLEEP WHEN SHE SLEEPS!

As you leave the hospital with your prem baby, here are some things which <u>developmental follow-ups will need to include:</u>

- ► regular weight checks;
- ► head circumference measurements;
- ► a developmental assessment every six months;
- ► regular hearing and eye examinations;
- ► check-ups with a speech therapist.

Your prem may need some physiotherapy help, especially in the first three years.

Some countries have "early intervention programmes" to follow up babies that have been born prematurely. Join these if you can.

<u>Things to be aware of</u>.

- ► Does your baby turn her head towards light and sound?
- ► Does your baby move her head if you hold a bright object and move it from side to side?
- ► Does she reach for things with both hands?

Ask you doctor or physiotherapist for daily exercises to do with your prem to strengthen her muscles and help her to develop "normally". Remember that the more little things you do early in her life, the more impact they will have. Do spend this time helping your baby, especially in the first few months and years. It will be the best investment of time that you could ever make.

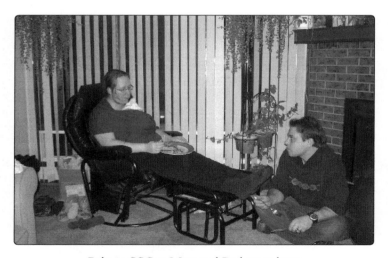

Baby in SSC as Mum and Dad are at home.

PARENTING

This chapter applies for every baby, but even more so for a sensitive baby. Prems are more likely to be sensitive.

There are many good books on parenting in the resources section, but you may not have time to read them now. Some books may be out of date and give advice which will not work for your baby.

Based on science, here are some important things to do (1). A lot of this is also "common sense", but some of these things seem to have been forgotten in western society and lost in technology.

Trust your instincts! (2)

If your baby cries, your natural reaction will be to pick her up and comfort her. This is the right reaction, so ignore the books that say "train her to sleep by leaving her to cry". There is no science to support their arguments.

Breastfeed:

Parents who carry their babies in skin-to-skin contact are more likely to breast feed their babies and breast feed for much longer with all the huge benefits (3). The American Academy of paediatrics recommends breastfeeding for two years (4). The skin-to-skin contact stimulates the release of prolactin and oxytocin hormones which help in breast milk production.

Bonding:

Babies need to belong! If Mum and baby have bonded well in the first hours and days and weeks of life, this will make it easier for your baby to trust and bond with others. "Attachment parenting" works because of basic biology, which happens because of skin-to-skin contact (1;5). Your baby on your chest at birth starts the hormones in you and your baby working together in the right way. This makes good parenting so much easier. You respond to your baby and give her what she needs.

When your baby is in the right place on your chest, she will have the "right" behaviour of stable heart rate and breathing, breastfeeding, sleeping and waking in a regular rhythm, absorbing food maximally, and bonding with you. Human babies are born with a strong urge to self-regulate. If she is born prematurely, your baby will need your help to regulate, and your body can automatically calm her. Babies are also born with a deep inner drive to bond, belong and communicate with Mum. Skin-to-skin contact helps these natural drives (as well as mothers' natural drive to protect and provide for her baby).

Some parents may be reading this book and feel guilty that they did not give their prem early skin-to-skin contact. You may have been in a NICU that did not understand the importance of this early bonding time. It is never too late to make contact with your baby or child. Lots of love and hugs, eye contact, focused listening to them and playing with them on their level can make your child feel more secure. Sitting reading to a bigger child with your arm around her will make a difference to her self-esteem.

Holding and carrying:

Holding and carrying your baby skin-to-skin will allow your newborn to experience the outside world from a safe place (6). Babies like to feel contained and be held quiet and still. This helps bonding and also encourages the mother to carry and hold her child for the first two years of life. This is what babies need for best brain-wiring and emotional security. This is particularly important during the first six to eight weeks for the part of the brain called the amygdala, which controls emotions. Carrying the baby is still very important after eight weeks. If you have twins, Dad, Granny or an aunt can carry a twin skin-to-skin. However, for the best effects for breastfeeding it would need to be mother, so each twin has a turn on mum.

Babies love to be carried.
Hold and carry for 1st 2 years.

Carrying the full term baby skin-to-skin can be done with any sling. When carrying a premature baby it is essential to stabilize the baby's airway. A KangaCarrier® will do this.

Tight swaddling and loud noises ("shushing") may get a baby to sleep, but possibly by her being too frightened to react. This may do long term harm to the baby and should be avoided.

Talk gently to her. It is worth investing time looking at your baby, playing with her and making eye-to-eye contact (1). It is important for Dad to spend time doing this too. (Remember that your prem may easily be over-stimulated and so start to focus elsewhere. Respect that and give her a break.)

Talk with your baby:

Talk to your baby to help make the best brain connections. Reading to your baby and young child has huge benefits. Singing and playing music has an organising effect on brain function.

Get involved:

Guard your baby's sense of security. Be careful not to let your newborn tiny baby be held by too many people. She feels safest with your familiar voices and smells

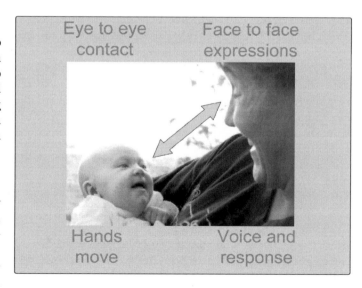

giving her security. You also want to reduce the risk of infections. If your baby's crying is prolonged when she is left at crèche or day care centre, consider investing time in your child's long term security by being at home with her for a while longer. Work will still be there in several months! It is the best investment of time you will ever make in your life! "Being there" applies for toddlers as well. If they are held close, then allowed of their own accord to go off to someone else, and come back to check that mum is still there, then go out again, they will be much more trusting, secure and confident.

> **BE there for your child. Babies spell LOVE as T-I-M-E.**

BEING there for your children is important for all ages. (It still applies when they are teenagers!) Being there means your interested and active involvement as well as time and love.

Time and love:

You cannot "spoil "a baby till 2–3 years. You cannot "over-love" a baby. But you can certainly "damage "a baby by loving it too little (7)!

Babies do take time! There are no short-cuts to love. In our fast-paced society, slowing down to BE present with your baby, will help your baby and will help you set more balanced priorities in your own life. Your baby is an individual person and needs to be respected as such, and talked to and listened to. Do fill up your baby's emotional tank by allowing her "cuddle time" and nurture her properly. The benefits will last a lifetime! <u>Play</u> with your baby as she grows. Play puts together all of the touch, eye contact, laughter and movement that are essential for brain wiring. In neuroscience, play is building the circuits to prepare for adult life.

Co-sleeping:

The debates around co-sleeping are endless. What is known is that babies benefit enormously from that close physical contact with their mothers. Sleep cycling is critical for brain wiring, and good sleep cycling only takes place in mother's presence. Babies in skin-to-skin contact do not sink into the deep apnoea sleep in which they stop breathing (this may cause SIDS or cot death).

Just as we drive a car safely with seatbelts, so co-sleeping must be done safely with no drugs, no smoking, no loose duvets, a firm pillow and a firm mattress (8). A cot next to your bed allows your arm to reach your baby in her own bed.

It has been suggested that working parents who have their babies in a crèche, can have their babies sleeping in their beds and this makes a big difference to the child's stability.

Note well – if mother or father is a smoker and co-sleeps with their infant, there is an increased risk of SIDS!

Different intelligences

We have written this book specifically about protecting and stimulating your baby's brain. Each sensation has its own intelligence or wiring (9). Please remember there are lots of different ways in which people are "intelligent" or gifted.

Learn and boost what your own baby is good at to build her self esteem. Encourage her with things that she struggles with. Some children are good at sport, some love music, art or languages. Those who are not good at these can still enjoy them! Some children are very good with people. Others prefer playing with numbers, others like building things in 3D. Encouraging all parts of a child will help her to grow up well-rounded and to reach her full potential as an individual.

Parenting twins and multiples

Twins and triplets have a higher risk of being born early so prems can also be multiples! That makes the first weeks and months at home even more of a challenge! Mothers of twins often say that you should wake the other twin when the first twin wakes, to try to get them feeding at the same time to protect your sleep (10;11).

If your twins are premature, place them together in an incubator for comfort facing each other. Better still place them together on your chest in skin-to-skin contact.

Ask for help from family and friends! Be aware that caring for twins can also be an added stress on your relationship.

Your decisions to act on:

....

....

....

....

....

....

....

Parenting specifically for prems

This whole book has been about this topic!!

To summarize:

For the first few weeks, skin-to-skin contact, mother's presence, breastfeeding, containment and a quiet environment are very helpful. Baby should be kept in flexion (legs and arms bent). Protect her sleep. Infant massage can be helpful. Do not leave her to cry.

In the first months,

Continue as above. Hold your baby and hug her lots. If you are reading this when your prem has grown a bit, it is never too late to give them extra hugs! Carry her as much a possible; she will sleep best this way! She will feel safe, and this will help her catch up her development.

Look after her sleep and do not wake her unnecessarily. Play with her when she is awake and start reading stories and singing songs

Watch your baby to see how much stimulation she can cope with. Try not to overwhelm her.

Start with small doses of stimulation and read her signals. Be sensitive to her. Hold a bright object above your baby's face. Move it from side to side to see if her eyes will follow it.

It is important for your baby to crawl, so from about three months of age put her down to lie on her tummy on the floor when she is awake for playing. She will start to lift her head and try to push herself up. This will strengthen upper body muscle tone. When she is sleeping, she can be on her back or side.

Avoid using walking rings for your baby. They do not help upper body tone and balance and they force her legs to move at an unnatural angle.

Here are some practical things for you as a parent to do, or look out for.

▷ Check that your prem responds to sounds; if a door slams by mistake and she does not react at all, it may be worth checking her hearing.

▷ Is your baby's body floppy if you hold her hands and pull her from lying to sitting position? When she is six months, can she sit? Does she usually fall over to the same side?

▷ Try to encourage her to use both arms and both legs equally. Try to keep her supple by gentle exercises like bicycling with her legs and arms as you play with her.

▷ Remember that she will need a lot of sleep and quiet play.

▷ It is important to have regular checkups. These will pick up possible problems early on, when it is much easier to work with them. Follow the advice your hospital gives you. If you are worried about anything, ask at your regular check ups. Prems have a lot to catch up and it may take time to do this. Go gently with them; be grateful and celebrate small progress.

> **Do NOT expect them to do all the things at the same age as a full term baby can.**

Fine Print Page – Parenting

1. This excellent Dorling Kindersley book covers parenting from birth to teenage years.
2. This short book summarises evidence on the key role mothers play in child development. The book can be downloaded free from the internet, link at bottom of page, http://www.imhaanz.org.nz/peter-cooks-mothering-denied-available-internet.
3. Biological Nurturing is based on the same neuroscience described in this book. Skin-to-skin contact and breastfeeding impact all aspects of good development. http://www.biologicalnurturing.com/
4. Given the conservative medical culture of the USA, the recommendation of the AAP reflects the strength of the evidence now available.
5. This article from Mothering" magazine may be easier to read than some of the scientific references here.
6. Book now available from http://www.hale-publishing.com/
7. A practical and helpful little book.
8. Co-sleeping is controversial, and McKenna explains the issues in away that is based on a broader and better understanding of the science. See website: http://www.nd.edu/~jmckenn1/lab/   Article can be downloaded from http://www.naturalchild.org/james_mckenna/cosleeping.pdf
9. Book may be challenging reading, but there are succinct summaries available on internet: http://www.davesabine.com/Music/Articles/MITheoryHowardGardner/tabid/170/Default.aspx
10–11. … two good books on managing twins at home !

Reference List

(1) Sunderland M. The Science of Parenting. Dorling Kindersley Limited, London; 2006.
(2) Cook P. Mothering denied. 2008.
(3) Colson S. Biological nurturing. Biological Nurturing 2005.
(4) American Academy of Pediatric : Section on Breastfeeding. Breastfeeding and the use of human milk. American Academy of Pediatrics 2005;115(2):496-506.
(5) Porter LL. The science of attachment: The biological roots of love. Mothering 2003 July;(119).
(6) Blois M. Babywearing. Pharmasoft Publishing, L.P.; 2005.
(7) Contey C, Takikawa D. CALMS A guide to soothing your baby. Hana Peace Works, Los Olivos; 2007.
(8) McKenna JJ, McDade T. Why babies should never sleep alone. A review of the co-sleeping controversy in relation to SIDS, bedsharing and breast feeding. Paediatric Respiratory reviews 2005;6:134-1.
(9) Gardner HE. Frames of Mind: The Theory of Multiple Intelligences. New York: Basic Books; 1983.
(10) Gromada KK. Mothering Multiples. Third ed. , USA: La Leche League International; 1999.
(11) Noble E. Having Twins - and more. Houghton Mifflin Company; 2003.

COMPASSIONATE CARE FOR A DYING BABY

This is a really hard section and my heart goes out to parents in this situation.

Many people avoid talking about death, but it is important.

A baby represents new life and a future, the opposite of death. So it is the "wrong way round" to watch a baby die so early.

If your baby is dying:

Many parents have been allowed to do skin-to-skin contact with their tiny baby even if she is dying. This is called compassionate care. (1). These parents have hugely valued being able to hold their tiny baby for the short time that they had together.

Adults do not want to die alone.
Do not leave your tiny baby to die alone.

Sometimes death occurs after weeks of struggling. Hold your baby as she dies. Give her permission to let go and stop struggling.

Give her a name; she is a real person and already has her own personality. It will help you, her parents to grieve her death appropriately.

If your baby has already died you may want to hold her to say goodbye. This can be important for you. Be aware that she may have a different skin colour and be cold.

Collect mementos such as a lock of hair and her tiny armband from the hospital.

Take photos of her, This will help you to treasure the memory of your very real baby.

If your tiny prem dies it may be an intense shock for you and you may have extremely strong reactions of grief. All of these are normal reactions, so don't fear that you are going mad. Your feelings may include sadness, anger, guilt, anxiety, helplessness, fatigue, relief. You may be physically numb, have tightness in your throat, lack energy, feel weak and be over-sensitive to noise. You may not believe that your baby has died or be confused. You may want to withdraw, lose your appetite, struggle to sleep, dream of your baby, sigh, cry and feel restless

▶ Do have a proper funeral – this allows you to mourn and grieve properly, and friends and family will support you.

▶ Don't try to pretend your baby did not exist (2).

▶ Get help from professionals / support groups (3).

▶ Be aware of the risk of depression.

You may find yourself "searching", yearning for your lost one (3;4). You cannot forget your baby or replace her. You may grieve for different lengths of time from your partner, feel anger and want to blame someone.

Feelings of wanting to get back into normal life and reinvesting in life are sometimes very slow to come and may take months. Allow this time of grieving and emotional ups and downs or waves.

It is important to be very careful how you tell small siblings. Siblings may have had to cope with Mum being away in hospital for weeks with the prem baby and may feel very rejected and jealous of the baby who was getting all the attention. If the baby dies, they may blame themselves because they were jealous of the baby.

Do be aware that if you have another pregnancy later, you may find yourself very anxious that this baby too may not survive. This is often overlooked. (4;5). Friends, family and medical staff will need to be extra supportive.

If you have a faith community or church, let the members support you. Be gentle with yourself. You have had a major life shock.

Fine Print Page – Compassionate Care.

1. This is one of the earliest recorded cases, and the skin-to-skin contact was an important aspect. The parents were obviously also supported in many other ways.
2. Staff often find it difficult – even after training – to talk to bereaved parents. These authors … "offer this column as a vehicle for reflecting on the meanings of words used during this particular time of loss and grief."
3. This review article describes 19 publications on perinatal bereavement or distressing birth experience counseling. Quote: 'Counseling strategies provided women with opportunities to talk about their birth experience, express feelings about what happened, have questions answered, address gaps in knowledge or understanding of events, connect the event with emotions and behavior, talk about future pregnancies, and explore existential issues." Conclusions about how effective these are cannot be drawn …, but that it is important is not questioned !!
4. A "Perinatal Bereavement Scale" is described, and it showed that "parents who have experienced a late perinatal loss (stillbirth or neonatal death) display more unresolved grief during a subsequent pregnancy and during the postnatal period than parents who have experienced a miscarriage."
5. This is a case report on a young mother with previous stillbirth, experiencing problems at the next birth, which resolve after starting skin-to-skin contact.

Reference List

(1) Collins S. Baby Stephanie: a case study in compassionate care. Neonatal Intensive Care 1993 March;6(2):47-9.
(2) Jonas-Simpson C, McMahon E. The Language of Loss When a Baby Dies Prior to Birth: Cocreating Human Experience. Nursing Science Quarterly 2005 April;18(2):124-30.
(3) Gamble J, Creedy D. Content and Processes of Postpartum Counseling After a Distressing Birth Experience: A Review. Birth: Issues in Perinatal Care 2004 September;31(3):213-8.
(4) Theut SK, Pedersen FA, Zaslow MJ, Cain RL, Rabinovich BA, Morihisa JM. Perinatal loss and parental bereavement. The American Journal Of Psychiatry 1989 May;146(5):635-9.
(5) Burkhammer MD, Anderson GC, Sheau-Huey C. Grief, Anxiety, Stillbirth, and Perinatal Problems: Healing With Kangaroo Care. JOGNN: Journal of Obstetric, Gynecologic, & Neonatal Nursing 2004 November;33(6):774-82.

RESOURCES

There is a huge amount of information on the internet and in the bookshops, with confusing advice! This is a very small selection of further information that is in line with the information in this manual, and which we recommend. There is a lot more very good information, there is also some which is not so helpful!

DVD / Videos:

By Jill and Nils Bergman:
Restoring the Original Paradigm for infant care and breastfeeding
Rediscover the Natural Way to care for your baby
Available at *www.kangaroomothercare.com*

By Christina Smillie: *Baby-led Breastfeeding*
By Dr Lennart Righard: *Delivery Self Attachment*
Available at *www.geddesproduction.com*
By Debby Takikawa: *What babies want*

Key websites:

NICU Care

www.kangaroomothercare.com	Skin-to-skin contact
www.prematurity.org	Information on NICU
www.nicuparentsupport.org	NICU parent support
www.compassionatefriends.org	Grief support
http://www.missfoundation.org	When a Child Dies
http://www.missingangelsbill.org	Stillbirth Policy Advocacy

Breastfeeding support

www.breastfeeding.com	
www.lalacheleague.org	
www.ilca.org	
www.hmbana.org	Human milk bank association of North America
www.geddesproduction.com	

Other resources

www.askdrsears.com	
www.babycentre.co.uk	
www.australianbabyhands.com	sign language for babies

Some helpful books to read

The Science of Parenting by Margot Sunderland, 2006. ISBN-13: 978-1-4053-1486-2.

Kangaroo Care: The best you can do to help your preterm infant by Susan Ludington-Hoe, Bantam Books, 1993.

Breastfeeding made simple by Nancy Mohrbacher, 2005. ISBN 1-57224-404-6.

When pregnancy follows a loss by Joann O'Leary. 2006. ISBN-13-978-0-9789439-0-5.

Fathers-to-be handbook by Patrick Houser, available http://fatherstobe.org/

CALMS: a guide to soothing your baby by Carrie Contey, Debby Takikawa http://calmsguide.com/

Come home soon, Baby brother by Debi Iarussi (A colouring in book for siblings of prems)

Sleeping with your baby by James Mc Kenna, Platypus Media.

Bonding by M. Klaus, J Kennell and P.Klaus.

Your amazing newborn by M. Klaus and P. Klaus, Perseus Books.

Why love Matters by Sue Gerhardt, Routledge, Taylor and Francis.

Biological Nurturing: laid-back breastfeeding by Dr Suzanne Colson, available from www.geddesproduction.com

Sweet Dreams: A pediatrician's secrets for your child's good night's sleep by Dr Paul Fleiss, Lowell House, Illinois.

Best medicine: Human milk in the NICU by Drs. Nancy Wight, Jane Morton, and Jai Kim. Hale Publishing.

Gentle Birth, Gentle Mothering by Dr Sarah Buckley, One Moon Press Brisbane Australia.

From the author

Thank you to the many people who have helped to make this book happen:

- the parents of premature babies who shared deeply with me; their experiences will help other parents who now have to walk this road;
- the parents who let us take photos of them and their babies;
- the nurses, doctors, developmental specialists and researchers who are so dedicated to premature babies and their parents;
- Peter Hartmann for permission to use his thermal image on page 50;
- Louise Goosen for letting me use a number of her photographs;
- Hilary Palser for her faithful encouragement in walking me through this book;
- Agneta Kleberg and Welma Lubbe, for insights on developmental care;
- Bronwyn Lusted and Ann Westoby for their diagrams;
- Paddy O'Leary my insightful and patient editor;
- Barbara Mueller for being such an encouragement in typesetting and bringing this book to completion.

My great thanks go to my husband Nils for all of his 20 years of holding onto his vision for improving the start for premature babies. He has distilled this broad-based knowledge from thousands of articles. He has continuously encouraged me to "translate" the medical jargon into everyday English for every parent. What a privilege to have such a wonderful husband, work partner and friend!

Above all, thank you Jesus, for the miracle of life and for being my SAFE place.